JEWISH VALUES IN HEALTH AND MEDICINE

Edited by

Rabbi Levi Meier, Ph.D.

Cedars-Sinai Medical Center
Los Angeles, California

Contributions

by

Immanuel Jakobovits

Maurice Lamm

Milton Heifetz

Miriam Lippel

David M. Feldman

William Cutter

Fred Rosner

Robert E. Levine

Levi Meier

David Hartman

J. David Bleich

Harold M. Schulweis

H.J.C. Swan

University Press
of America

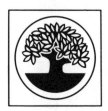

Lanham • New York • London

Copyright © 1991 by
University Press of America®, Inc.
4720 Boston Way
Lanham, Maryland 20706

3 Henrietta Street
London WC2E 8LU England

Library of Congress Cataloging-in-Publication Data

Jewish values in health and medicine / edited by Levi Meier.
p.   cm.
Includes bibliographical references and index.
1. Medical ethics.   2. Ethics, Jewish.
3. Sick—Psychology—Case studies.
R725.57.J493 1990
296.3'85642—dc20   90–23835 CIP

ISBN 0–8191–8173–0 (cloth)
ISBN 0–8191–8174–9 (paper)

Dedicated

in Honor of

Blanche Salick

CONTENTS

PART III
CLINICAL ISSUES

CONTRIBUTORS

RABBI J. DAVID BLEICH, Ph.D.
Professor of Talmud
Yeshiva University, New York

Professor of Law
Benjamin Cardozo School of Law, New York

RABBI WILLIAM CUTTER, Ph.D.
Professor of Education
Hebrew Union College
Los Angeles, California

RABBI DAVID M. FELDMAN, D.H.L.
Former Chairman
Committee on Medical Ethics
Federation of Jewish Philanthropies, New York

RABBI DAVID HARTMAN, Ph.D.
President, Hartman Institute
Jerusalem, Israel

MILTON HEIFETZ, M.D.
Neurosurgeon
Cedars-Sinai Medical Center
Los Angeles, California

LORD IMMANUEL JAKOBOVITS, Ph.D.
Chief Rabbi
The British Commonwealth of Nations

RABBI MAURICE LAMM, D.D.
President
National Institute for Jewish Hospice
Los Angeles, California

ROBERT E. LEVINE, M.D.
Professor of Clinical Ophthalmology
University of Southern California School of Medicine

Fellow, American Society of Ophthalmic Plastic and Reconstructive Surgery

MIRIAM LIPPEL, M.A.
Director
Coalition for Advancement of Jewish Education (CAJE) Curriculum Bank
Los Angeles, California

RABBI LEVI MEIER, Ph.D.
Chaplain
Cedars-Sinai Medical Center
Los Angeles, California

Psychologist in private practice

FRED ROSNER, M.D.
Director, Department of Medicine
Queen's Hospital Medical Center, New York

Professor of Medicine
State University of New York, Stony Brook

RABBI HAROLD M. SCHULWEIS, Th.D.
Valley Beth Shalom
Encino, California

H.J.C. SWAN, M.D., Ph.D.
Professor of Medicine
University of California, Los Angeles
School of Medicine

Former Director of Cardiology
Cedars-Sinai Medical Center
Los Angeles, California

THE MAX MARTIN SALICK MEMORIAL LECTURESHIP

Dedicated in Honor of Blanche Salick

Blanche Salick is the matriarch of the Salick family. She honored the memory of her husband by being a sponsor of the first series of Max Martin Salick lectures published in 1986. Her fortitude and patience through years of hardship resulted in the success not only of her children, but of a whole generation of family members.

In 1934, as a young bride and immigrant, she set up a home on the Lower East Side of New York and started working in the family laundry business. She had to adjust to the difficulties of this new life, which was very different from what she had known in her comfortable, traditional home in her native Rumania. Her new home was Jewish in every respect, and she tried to maintain the same spiritual and religious commitment that she was taught. In a single communication at the end of the War in 1945, she learned that her parents, four of her sisters, her brother and many other family members had perished as saintly martyrs of the Holocaust.

Turning despair into constructive action, she made her home into a rehabilitation center for the surviving relatives, many of whom were distant and many of whom had to be expatriated at great expense and difficulty. Her spirit, encouragement and selfless nurturing gave many a new start and a hope for the future. She became a bedrock of support for those trying to put their lives together.

Now, some forty years later, many have achieved wonderful successes and they have flourished. They live all across this continent, as well as in the State of Israel. All are productive citizens.

All her children, grandchildren, cousins, nieces, nephews, sisters and extended family members love her dearly and respect her contribution to our well-being and to the cohesiveness of the Salick family. We dedicate this book to her eternal optimism and to the spirit and love and support that she has provided us all.

The Salick Family

THE SALICK FAMILY

Members of the Salick family are pictured with the guest lecturers at the 10th Annual (1989) Max Martin Salick Memorial Lectureship in Jewish Medical Ethics. Seated are Mrs. Blanche Salick, wife of the late Max Martin Salick, and Allen Salick, M.D. Standing are (l-r) Gloria Salick, Bernard Salick, M.D., Renee Salick, Ed.D., Rabbi Levi Meier, Ph.D., Fred Rosner, M.D., Candace Salick and Cedars-Sinai Scientific Director, Charles Kleeman, M.D.

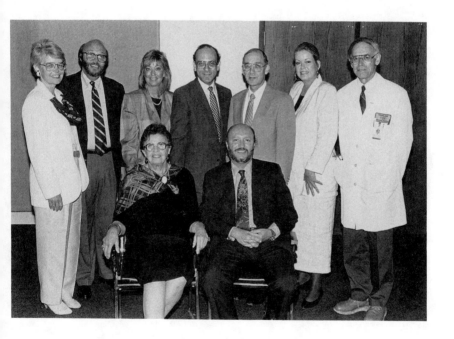

ACKNOWLEDGEMENTS

It is with a great deal of gratitude that I acknowledge the assistance that I have received in the preparation of this book.

I would like to thank Paula Van Gelder, Assistant to the Chaplaincy Department, who in her expert professional and creative manner, critically read the manuscript and enhanced the styles of the various authors. I would also like to thank Faith Joy Dantowitz for carefully proofreading the entire text and Gita Fuchs for preparing the manuscript in camera-ready format.

The family of Max Martin Salick, particularly Blanche Salick to whom this book is dedicated, has encouraged, supported and facilitated the annual lectureships on Jewish medical ethics in memory of Max Martin Salick. I cherish their friendship.

The staff of the word processing center -- Joye L. Nunn-Hill, Denise M. Kurushima and Chris Collier -- and my former secretary, Josie Bonorris, deserve recognition for their devoted service in the production of this work.

I would like to express my appreciation to the Board of Rabbis of Southern California, specifically to Rabbi Martin Ryback, Director of Chaplaincy, and Rabbi Paul Dubin, Executive Vice President, and to the Jewish Federation Council of Greater Los Angeles for cooperating in our mutual endeavors.

I would like to thank the Administration, Board of Directors and Board of Governors of Cedars-Sinai Medical Center for having the vision and foresight to include the spiritual component, pastoral counseling and medical ethical issues as part of the overall health care approach involved in the recovery of patients.

My appreciation is also expressed to Steve Broidy, Founding Life Chairman of Cedars-Sinai Medical Center; Robert L. Spencer and Ernest J. Friedman, consecutive Chairmen of the Board of Directors; Frieda Meltzer, Life Trustee; Sheldon King, President, and his predecessor, Stuart J. Marylander; Larry Baum, Vice President for Community Relations; Thomas Priselac, Executive Vice President; and Dr. Michael Langberg, Director, Department of Medical Education, who have, with professionalism and dedication, contributed to the spiritual well-being of patients and their families at Cedars-Sinai Medical Center.

I would also like to express my gratitude to the patients, physicians and nurses who have consulted me and opened their hearts to discuss difficult issues.

I wish to also pay tribute to my mentor, Dr. James Kirsch, of blessed memory, who helped me focus on each individual patient's experience.

Another mentor, Dr. Manfred Altman, of London, England, has constantly served as a source of inspiration to me.

My father, Alfred Meier, of blessed memory, and my mother, Frieda Meier, have always served as exemplary models to me.

Finally, of course, I acknowledge the loving support of my dear wife, Marcie, and our four children -- Chana, Yosef Asher, Malka Mindel and Yitzchak Shlomo -- who have created a beautiful and warm atmosphere that facilitated the completion of this work.

INTRODUCTION

The subject matter of Part I -- the clinical experiences of patients -- was specifically selected as the first portion of this work. Ultimately, all theories of medical ethics must be applied to the experiences of patients, and to their individual perspectives, both in sickness and in health. It is my privilege to present chapters by Miriam Lippel, Rabbi William Cutter and Rabbi Harold Schulweis that deal with personal experiences during illness, surgery and a near-death state.

Part II, dealing with the foundation of Jewish medical ethics, follows the experiences of patients and their families. This section presents essential aspects of the Jewish heritage, based on Biblical, Rabbinic and other Jewish sources of the past 2,000 years. The aim of this section is cohesiveness and a presentation of clear guidelines. Dr. Robert E. Levine, Dr. Milton Heifetz, Dr. David Hartman, Dr. Fred Rosner, Rabbi Maurice Lamm and I have presented some fundamental guidelines, based on Jewish values, concerning basic principles of Jewish medical ethics, human dignity in the physician-patient relationship, the role and responsibilities of the physician and the Jewish component in hospice care.

Part III of this book deals with clinical issues. It is recommended that the reader compare and contrast the contents of Part I, patients' experiences, with the clinical issues discussed in Part III by prominent Rabbis, ethicists, physicians and other scholars. Dr. Fred Rosner and Rabbi J. David Bleich deal with some general concerns in their respective chapters on ethical dilemmas in medical practice and care of the terminally ill. Specific, contemporary issues are then addressed by Rabbi David M. Feldman (Baby M) and Dr. Fred Rosner (Jewish perspectives on AIDS). Central to all patient concerns is the exploration of why a specific illness has happened to them at a particular time in their lives. In reflecting on this universal experience, Dr. Jeremy Swan and I clarify the poignancy and centrality of this issue, as we look at this process of exploration as part of the healing process. We are indebted to Chief Rabbi Immanuel Jakobovits for his probing and thought-provoking analysis and discussion of the human reaction to illness and misfortune.

The reader can clearly compare and contrast subjective patient experiences with objective discussions of clinical issues. Reading all of this material together leads one to the conclusion that Jewish values and guidelines are just that -- guidelines. People need to be educated to understand these underlying concepts, yet the patient's experience is so private and personal that no stethoscope can pick up every internal tick and sigh. The patient's decision needs to be respected so that ultimately, it will serve as a new guideline for future generations.

FOREWORD

By publishing a variety of well-researched writings on medical and health issues in the light of Jewish teachings, Rabbi Levi Meier has established himself as a widely-recognised writer in this field.

In contrast to many others now contributing to the significant development of this relatively new discipline, our author adds to his considerable academic knowledge years of practical experience in pastoral care and moral counselling.

It is this combination of practice and theory which lends this work, as others produced by him, a specially topical appeal, of interest to lay readers as well as to specialists.

I hope this volume will further enhance understanding and respect for Jewish teachings in an area of increasing importance for the preservation of moral values and their supremacy over technological advances.

Lord Jakobovits
Chief Rabbi

PART I

PATIENTS' EXPERIENCES

CHAPTER 1

RECOLLECTION OF THE HEART--

A PERSONAL MEMOIR

Miriam Lippel, M.A.

The first time I sat down with pen and paper to begin telling the story of my heart surgery I found myself staring blankly at the white sheet, feeling as blank as the paper in front of me. There was so much to say, so much to tell, so much, in fact, that I felt helpless to even begin. Could I possibly confront all the confusing and intense emotions that still reside within me? And once having confronted them, could I possibly accurately communicate them? And what was it I wanted to communicate anyway? I decided ultimately that it was not necessary for me to justify my need to express what happened to me or how it made me feel, but that the expression had meaning in and of itself. It is meaningful to me and if it is meaningful to others, then it shall have been all the more worth the effort it took to open my heart (pun intended) and relate it.

Despite my good intentions, I was still blocked. So I went to the beach, my favorite think place. I watched the waves and let myself be lulled by the rhythm of the surf as it hit the shore. I remembered suddenly that one of the ways I coped with the physical pain of my surgery was by imagining that I was body surfing. Pain, too, has its rhythms and the trick was to sense its ebb and flow and to float above it, to catch the peak and ride with it until it rested you weakly on the shore. Of course, there were always waves that caught me by surprise and smashed me gasping onto the beach, but that was to be expected. Practice makes perfect, however, and there was enough pain for me to learn the skill quite well.

Somehow, that memory started me thinking; I found myself comparing life to the ocean. It has rhythms and cycles, it is sometimes calm, sometimes stormy. It is mysterious, known and yet unknown. We hold at the same moment delight in its splendor and terror at its uncharted depths. As I watched the sunset there on the beach I felt a togetherness with the universe and a terrible aloneness at the same time. I wondered about the nature of God and how my thinking about and experience of God and religion had changed. I thought of life and death, of despair and hope, of joy and sorrow, of illness and health, and began to feel the oneness of all those seeming opposites; to confront one meant to acknowledge the other. You can learn about one by learning about the other. With those thoughts in mind, I was finally able to sit down and relive on paper the experiences that I will now share with you. This narrative reflects the struggle, anger, ambivalence and confusions that arose during that period of my life but I hope that it also affirms my love of life and gratefulness to those who helped preserve it and who have loved me through the healing process.

The First Five Days

In July of 1986, I was a full-time graduate student in Jewish education at the University of Judaism, holding down two or three part-time jobs depending on the day of the week, and in the process of moving into a new apartment. I did not have time to be sick. Besides, I was not in the habit of giving in to every little symptom I felt. Nevertheless, when I began to have symptoms that appeared to be developing into a serious bronchial infection I went to my doctor. I had a low fever, fatigue, a dry cough and some mild breathing problems when I exerted myself. I also had night sweats which I attributed to the fever, as well as swollen ankles which I attributed to water retention from my period. I and my doctor were convinced that I was pushing myself too hard and that I had a bronchial infection. I did not look that sick; I did not sound very sick. You would never have known from looking at me, a healthy-appearing 25-year-old woman, that I was having congestive heart failure. That was something old people have, right? Anyway, I did what the doctor ordered and religiously stayed in bed for a week but did not get any better. In fact, I seemed to be getting worse. I had to sleep sitting up because lying down made me feel as though I was drowning. My ankles got very swollen, as did my waistline, and I began to have diarrhea and other digestive problems.

I hope you will forgive the indelicacy of this revelation but during one unpleasant trip to the bathroom at this time, I experienced my very first California earthquake. My first thought as the walls rattled around me was that somehow my bowel distress had messed up the Los Angeles sewer system. I remember laughing with relief when my roommate came running into my room to confirm that this had indeed been an earthquake and not a case of catastrophic flatulence!

After two return visits to my physician, a chest x-ray revealed that my heart was enlarged. I was sent immediately to Cedars-Sinai Medical Center for some tests to determine what was going on. I was unhappy about having to go into the hospital and nervous that something was wrong with my heart, but the full impact of what was happening had not sunk in yet. I was admitted on a Friday afternoon. Two of my sisters, who happened to be here on vacation, accompanied me. Their presence was so helpful to me as I felt frightened and small being shuffled from one office to another in this huge hospital full of strangers.

There were all sorts of preliminary questionnaires and examinations. At moments, I felt like I was being given the third degree, that somehow I should know what was wrong with me and how I got it. As ridiculous as it sounds, I felt guilty for being sick and putting everyone through all this bother. On some level, I was still clinging to the idea that this was just a bronchial infection and no big deal. My clothes were taken away, I was placed in hospital gowns, and strange slippers were stuck on my feet. I gave my purse and a few small jewelry items to my sister for safekeeping. All of the external, personal trademarks that were signs of my identity were suddenly removed and replaced with a plastic ID bracelet on my wrist and on my ankle. It was a strange feeling.

The sun began to set and the latest in what seemed to be a constant stream of doctors was asking me some questions about what I did and who I was. This was the first time anybody wanted to know who I was independent of my symptoms. I told him where I went to school and what I was studying. When he heard I was studying Jewish education, he noted the setting sun and wished me a "good *Shabbos*" as he left. I appreciated the greeting even though it focused me on how unhappy I was about being there in the first place and that this was not going to be much of a *Shabbos*.

I had informed my parents about what was happening and my mother, sensing that this was more serious than I thought, flew to Los Angeles immediately. My father joined her later. As independent and self-sufficient as I am, this situation brought out the frightened child in me, and having my family near was a comfort and a source of strength and support. They diluted somewhat the feeling of detached isolation that kept creeping up on me. Later on, however, even having loved ones close did not mitigate the alienation I experienced. In fact, at times it was aggravated by their presence. I felt compelled to be brave and resolute most of the time because I could see the worry and concern in their faces and did not want to cause them more pain on my account. My family did the best they could to be there for me but I let no one breach my innermost core. It took a great deal of energy to be "nice" all the time, and there were moments when crying or screaming would have been a welcome release of energy and anger but I suppressed most of the rage, despair and loneliness, and kept a stiff upper lip. There were intense thoughts and dynamics constantly going on inside of me that had no outward expression, but they left their mark on my psyche and returned to haunt me later.

One example of this process occurred during a gynecological procedure in which some fluid was drawn from a mass in my lower abdomen that was suspected of being the source of the infection that had travelled to my heart. The only way to reach it was intravaginally. A little over a year before I had been sexually assaulted by a man I had been dating. I never told anybody about it. I was far from home, alone in a distant city; I blamed myself; I pretended it never happened. This gynecological procedure was the first time since that event that anybody had touched me genitally and even though I knew intellectually that this was different, that this was a doctor, that this was not violence, the emotional trauma that was going on inside my head was tremendous. The whole incident replayed itself in my mind; I wanted to scream but could not. I was trapped captive and alone in that memory. It was like being raped again. In both cases, I was just a body having something done to me, an object not a subject. The only way I could deal with what was happening to me was to detach my conscious mind from my body. I found myself "seeing" the backs of the doctor's and nurse's lab coats and the tops of their heads as if I were floating above them and not the patient below. Of course, I could tell no one without revealing all and I was unable to face doing that. I made more trauma for myself with my silence and in a sense allowed myself to be victimized once more.

By the end of the fourth day of my hospital stay, most of the important facts about my condition had been ascertained. I was suffering from bacterial endocarditis, with a massive vegetation of staphylococcus situated on my aortic valve. It was clear that I was going to require surgery, but there was concern that I was too weak to survive it. I was being treated with huge doses of antibiotics in hopes of stabilizing me to the point where surgery would be possible. My doctors were also concerned that the infection could break off and give me a stroke.

I knew basically what was wrong with me. I had been briefed by my doctor but the fact that I could actually die had not sunk in yet. It was not until I overheard a conversation between two of the medical personnel in the Intensive Care Unit (ICU), who were standing outside my room discussing my condition, that I realized how badly off I really was. I do not remember exactly what it was that they said but it was clear that they thought I was asleep and could not hear them. The gist of it was that a particular doctor was really worried that I was not going to make it and that chances were I would die during the surgery, if I actually got to that point at all.

I began to think about the things I had not had the chance to do yet, the dreams I wanted to accomplish. I had done a great many different things in my 25 years, more than most people my age and I was proud of them, but there were other things I always thought I would have the time to do. I was young, I did not need to hurry, right? I always wanted to write a great play, or a novel. I had never been to Israel, or England or Italy.

I was saddest about the fact that I had never had a fulfilling relationship with a man, no chance to marry or have children and now it seemed that I never would. I promised myself that I would really "live" if I survived all this and I would do all the things I wanted to. I did not want to die and resolved to keep fighting for my life no matter how hard it got.

I kept telling myself that I would get through this no matter what the doctors said, but overhearing that conversation was demoralizing. It would have been one thing if the seriousness of my condition had been discussed with me, but to overhear it, whispered in the doorway, made me frightened and furious.

I wondered if God was there and why this was happening to me. I could not think of anything I had done that was terrible enough to deserve this. In truth, my conception of God is not so simplistic nor one of cause and effect, yet the overwhelming feeling that I was being punished pervaded me. I felt that the much lauded, supposedly just and kind God had turned away from me and I was angry, so I turned away in response.

Anybody who represented God and religion to me became the object of my anger. I internally rejected anything ceremonial or traditional. It all seemed at that moment futile and ridiculous. I did not want to hear about anything Jewish, yet ironically, later, I was able to find healing, comfort, inspiration and meaning in the images and symbols that abound in Judaism. They did not work for me until I was ready to reach for them, however.

I did not feel comfortable talking to anybody about my religious turmoil, so I tried not to think about it too much. My energy needed to be put into breathing and concentrating on staying alive, but the anger still burned within me, unspoken.

Surgery

I seemed to be somewhat stable until the fifth day in the hospital. During the early hours of the morning on July 30th, I had a cardiac arrest. My memory of that evening is nightmarish. My diabetes was completely out of control, a situation that added to my discomfort. I kept going in and out of consciousness. I wrote a description of what that night was like in my journal several weeks afterwards. I will let it speak for me rather than try to recount all the specific details:

Last night. I remembered the last night - the night they stopped my heart to fix it. I can hear the sound of my breath catching, gasping. I feel like I am drowning but there is no water. Funny how I have the sensation of being pulled down and, yet, floating at the same time. So heavy and so light. I want to sink but the sounds of the beeping machines keep bringing my mind back to the edge of reality. The faces keep changing above me. They are lost in shadow, blurred beyond recognition. If only they would get close enough so I could see them and know who is there. It is hopeless without my glasses, everything is blurred like some macabre Impressionist painting. One face after another, voices talking above me, about me, but not to me.

Someone changes an IV. I am so tired I cannot even scream so I just absorb the pain. At least I know I am alive, although at this moment I would rather not be. Someone is pushing hard on my chest. It is agony. I keep wondering when my life is going to pass before my eyes, is not that what is supposed to happen before you die? I wait but it does not happen. I only see changing shadows, whirling colors, misty faces. The pressure in my chest gets worse, like some infernal incubus trying to take my soul by force. "I won't let you," I keep thinking but I do not know who I am talking to - myself or God. I want to cry but I cannot, it is all locked inside me, besides I do not have enough breath to cry. Once in a while my breath sounds to me like a *shofar* [ram's horn] with no sound.

I have no sense of time, minutes pass or hours, I cannot tell. Suddenly my mother is there and my Aunt Barbara. I cannot see their faces but I recognize their voices. Someone is getting me ready for surgery. They wash me and shave my body hair. I do not even have the energy to be embarrassed. Barbara (who is a nurse) is there and helping to prepare me for surgery so I am not so frightened. She is saying soothing things; so is the other nurse but I do not know what they are saying, I can only hear their tone of voice. I am trying to do what they want me to do but I can hardly move; every effort seems to be nearly impossible.

My mother is back. She says they are ready to take me to surgery. Her face is so scared but she is trying to give me courage. I suddenly realize that I have the strength to face whatever is next, so I tell her, "Don't worry about me, I'm going to make it." Not that I am sure at all about it, but at least my family will know I died hoping - not whimpering.

Halls are rushing past me. Every jostle of the gurney hurts but I say nothing. Words are no longer important to me. More rooms, blurred rooms, cold rooms, distant voices. Someone says: "This will just hurt for a second, sweetheart." Someone is looking in my eyes, their face is close to mine. They have brown eyes. Suddenly all the light is bright around me for a second and then the deepest darkness I have ever known.

Post-Op

I was awake very little during the 24 hours after my surgery, and what I remember most is the strange, disembodied heaviness I experienced. There were moments when I was aware of movement and sound around me, and the sensation of being touched. I had no urge to speak and no need to. I could sense time by the automatic blood pressure cuff that would inflate every fifteen minutes or so. It tightened against my upper arm with a strong grip and released with a strange hiss. The first feeling I was conscious of was the pulsing sensation it generated in my arm as it deflated.

As I began to be more alert the next day, I became aware of the temperature of the air around my body. It was cold. I could not move my head to see, and without my glasses it would have been a futile exercise anyway. My body did not feel like it was mine. My mind seemed to be working all right. I was talking to myself in my head a mile a minute--Can I feel my toes? Can I move my hands? What is happening? Where is my mother? Am I all right?

At some point my mother was in my room, standing by my bed and, being the verbal person that I am, I immediately wanted to talk. I had no idea, however, that I had a respirator in my throat. No one had explained that I would have one. I tried to tell my mother that I was cold. I thought I was telling her, anyway. But there was no response from her. I tried again. She seemed to be aware that I was talking but she obviously did not understand what I was saying. I tried desperately to communicate, but was unsuccessful. Then I thought perhaps I had had the stroke that the doctors had feared and that my brain was confused. Perhaps I was thinking one thing and saying another, or speaking gibberish. I kept trying. I felt tears of frustration welling up in my eyes and a terrible lump in my throat (which was probably the respirator tube but I did not know it). This was worse than death, to be trapped fully conscious in my body and unable to communicate anything. People would think I was hopeless, a vegetable, no one would know I was alive in here. I was thinking, hearing, screaming: "I'm still Miriam. Don't leave me, please. Listen, can't you hear me? I'm intelligent; I know what's going on! Help me!"

Waves of despair shook me to my very essence. I wanted to die at that moment if my fears were true. I prayed to God to be merciful and let me die; then I begged. I had one last test - I tried to spell "cold" using the manual alphabet for the deaf. As a teenager, I had attended some classes in sign language because I wanted to be able to talk to the two deaf children who lived across the street from me. I had forgotten most of the signs but I still remembered the alphabet. I weakly moved my left hand, spelling the word into the air. Even holding my arm up that far was a tremendous effort and it exhausted me. My mother looked at me, still confused. My heart sank in despair but I mustered the strength to try once more before giving up. At that moment the nurse happened to enter the room and stood next to me. She gave me an odd look as I waved my hand at her.

"I'm lost," I thought, "this is hopeless." Suddenly, she realized I was spelling. She took my hand and told me to try again. I slowly spelled c-o-l-d into her hand and she said the letters out loud as I spelled them. She got very excited and my mother looked so relieved. I felt so overwhelmed with gratefulness that I thought I would burst. The nurse brought me another blanket and I dozed off warm and thankful that I was not trapped in that living hell.

Near Death

The next day I had another brief arrest. I remember that I was sitting propped up in my bed. One of the nurses had just left the room after telling me something. Suddenly, I heard the heart monitor alarm go off right next to me. I turned my head to look at it and thought, "Oh, I wonder if my heart has stopped." Then I stopped breathing. I felt my body slump back on the pillows. I knew I stopped breathing and I knew there was nothing I could do about it. There was no struggle; in fact, I remember noting that the tremendous pain I was in was gone. It was a relief.

I was looking straight in front of me out the door of my ICU room and then my visual fields began to narrow and close in, like tunnel vision. It was as if I were being pulled backwards through a tunnel. The light of the room became a small dot in the distance and then disappeared altogether. I was not afraid, even though I was being propelled backwards through this long darkness; just curious, wondering what would be on the other end. I sensed that I was being drawn towards light but had not cleared the tunnel far enough to be in the midst of it yet. But then I felt my pace slow down, stop briefly, and begin to reverse itself. Now I was being pushed in the opposite direction, from where I had just come. A breeze brushed lightly against my face. I saw a pinhole of light in the distance that got larger and larger, and suddenly I was aware of the room around me, except now I was staring at the ceiling instead of the door. I knew something extraordinary had happened because the terrible pain that left the moment I entered the tunnel had now returned full force, and a terrible sense of sadness and regret flowed over me that I had come out on this side instead of the other.

I did not share my experience with anyone at first. I thought they would think I was crazy or hallucinating. And even now, though I am telling you about it, I cannot truly "share" it with you. To have come so close to death and returning to the source of my soul has left me with a knowledge and feelings that I cannot communicate. It is an emotion that is like none other. It has changed me in ways that I find difficult, if not impossible to articulate. It is the ultimate, personal experience and very private. I have had no fear of death since; in fact, there have been times when I have even yearned for it, at moments when struggling with life's difficulties seemed futile and overwhelming. I have, however, embraced the challenge and struggle of living, knowing full well that I will have the opportunity at some other time to go all the way through the tunnel.

I wrote a short poem not long after my hospital stay about some of the ambivalence I felt at having lived.

Thanatopsis--A Meditation on Death

I long to drink the waters of Lethe, to fade and
        float untethered to the world,
To evanesce like vapor,

Like my breath on a cold, winter morning,
Melding with the air unresisting,
To flow gently against the smiling cheek of a child
          on a summer's day,
To drift ethereal past pain, past fear, past lies
          and awesome truths.
I've looked Death in the face, drank tea in his parlor,
And am forever changed.
I know that I will face that brink again, the
          fearful precipice, enter its shadowy chasm
          another time, another moment. When?
Will I be ready then? I doubt it.
          Funny thing, how in one breath
          I can justify and, just, defy my death.

Recovery

It would be nice to report that after the surgery I bounced back into the bloom of health, but that is not the way it worked. My recovery was slow. It seemed interminable. It was complicated by my diabetes, kidney failure, digestive problems and fluid retention from heart failure, among other things. All told, I spent eight weeks in the hospital, eighteen days of which were in the Intensive Care Unit. Nor were those eight weeks restful recuperation. They were filled with shots, blood tests, physical therapy, IVs, pain and nightmares. There was so much to contend with physically and emotionally. Each day brought some new part of the battle to light.

There were many things to adjust to, any one of which would have been hard enough. On the outside, there was my scar, which seemed monstrous to me. For months after the surgery, all I would see when I looked into the mirror was the scar. I hated it. It took a long time for me not to be self-conscious about it and even now, two-and-one-half years later, there are times when I look at it and the memory of what it represents floods over me. Recently, in a reflective mood, I penned this hastily into my journal:

My scar is 10 and 1/2 inches long and runs down my chest,
    Right down the center,
Evenly spaced between my breasts where I once naively
    painted rouge so it would look like I had cleavage,
a sure sign of mature womanhood, I used to think
If only I had cleavage I would know everything
Or at the very least, appear as if I did.
I don't need to paint age on my body anymore,
Illness has done it for me.
Funny word that, cleavage. It means to be in the state of being split
    or cleft, a fissure or division. And so I am, a soul with deep
    chasms running here and there. Somehow, I think my incision
    is just an outward sign of what lies within. At times, when I
    look in the mirror, my scar looks to me like the angry crack
    pushed through the pavement of my street during the last
    earthquake. And at other times, I think it is a badge of
    courage that only those closest to me know about since it is
    hidden underneath my clothes. A tender heart lies underneath
    that scar, that has been bruised, that needs to heal and be
    nurtured; a heart that lives but knows every moment that it
    will die; a heart that yearns for a wholeness that seems elusive
    and mysterious.

My scar was only one new element to contend with. Even more
difficult than that was becoming accustomed to the sound of the artificial
heart valve that was used to replace my diseased one. The artificial heart
valve (St. Jude's model) makes a mechanical click every time it shuts. If
you are standing close to me in a quiet room you can hear it quite clearly.
I sound like a Timex! I came up with a whole host of "heart-valve" jokes
to describe my new condition. I told everyone that now I could rent my
body to terrorists as a timing device for dynamite. I was a natural to play
the ticking crocodile in "Peter Pan." The Los Angeles Philharmonic wanted
to use me as a metronome for their rehearsals. The only problem was that
in order to change my tempo they had to put me to sleep or get me excited.
The nurses thought I was hysterical. Sometimes, though, a laugh can be the
same as a cry.

I heard (and still hear) the ticking constantly. It was maddening, not
unlike the beating heart in Poe's classic horror story of "The Tell-Tale

Heart." It was an ever-present reminder of my mortality. I heard my existence ticking away all day and all night long. I would tune into the sound and feel emotionally paralyzed. It was as if my mind could not carry on the everyday business of life at the same moment that it was so acutely aware of death. Here is an entry from my journal written not long after I was discharged from the hospital:

> The clock in my room is silent, glowing blood red in the darkness with its LED numbers, as my heart ticks on marking the passage of ever-rushing time. Seconds lost, a constant reminder of life and death. I lie here frozen, watching different shades of darkness shift across the ceiling, grey, blue, green. I am lost in an abyss of swirling black, afraid to feel, afraid to trust myself or others. I do not know who I am anymore. I cannot find my masks or I do not have the energy to even look. I do not know how to just be or maybe I am just terrified of experiencing just being whoever I am without the comforting facades I hide behind. They give me structure and form; they are socially acceptable. People do not seem to see ME anymore; I am so afraid that all they will see is a heart problem and my scar. They will fear the illness and death that could be theirs if fate turns its evil side towards them as it has to me. I remind them that they are not invulnerable.

The constant thinking about death combined with daily concern over my condition was very stressful. My emotional state, as a result, was strained and erratic. It seemed that the better I got physically, the greater was the impact of what had actually happened to me. I had terrible paranoid nightmares filled with doctor zombies who were chasing me down the halls and nurses who were plotting to kill me. I also had a problem with memory.

It is not at all uncommon for people who have undergone major heart surgery to have short-term memory losses, as a result of the anesthesia and the heart and lung machine. It is a temporary condition but one that no one told me I might encounter. I found that I was forgetting what people had just said to me two minutes before. I could not remember who visited me that day sometimes, or who called. I had to write everything down and hope that I remembered to look at the piece of paper I had written it on. I felt constantly embarrassed by the fact that I kept forgetting things, and the uncomfortable reaction I got from some of my friends made it worse. I was afraid to ask about it, even though I knew there was something distinctly wrong. Afraid to get more bad news, I took a while to get up the nerve to ask my doctor. He said it would be temporary and he was right.

People's visits and comments all had great significance for me. I lived for when someone would walk through the door just to be with me. My friend, Judy, came nearly every day. On some days when I was too tired to talk, she just sat with me while I fell asleep. Seeing the face of a friend before I drifted off to sleep was comforting and reassuring to me, especially since I feared that I might never wake up again. The most amusing incident I remember was when a delivery man came to deliver a live tropical fish to the ICU! Some family friends sent it as a get-well present. It was hysterically funny. I asked the nurses to put it into the intravenous bag that hung above my bed, but they did not oblige. The fish went to stay with my cousins until such time as I could take care of it.

I taped all the get-well cards on the wall so that each morning I would remember that there were people who loved me and cared. I needed to know that all the time. The loneliness of being sick would creep in so fast, and the accompanying depression made each day a veritable emotional roller coaster. I coped by talking all the time, and making jokes. I thought I could fool everybody into thinking I was doing terrifically well, and in some ways I was, but there was so much unsaid and no one I felt safe enough to tell it to. Not even God.

God and I were not on speaking terms at that point. I was not even sure I believed in God anymore. And if there was a God, I wanted to sue for malpractice! Yes, yes, everyone told me, friends, relatives, doctors, what a miracle it was that I was alive, and how grateful I should be for being that way. And truthfully, I was grateful, but I was more angry and unhappy than grateful. The last thing I wanted was to have people tell me how lucky I was, and how it could have been worse. I did not feel lucky at all; I perceived my future and experienced my present as one continuous, painful and lonely struggle.

One night when I was experiencing some extreme abdominal discomfort and was in a lot of pain, one of the nurses tried to convert me to Christianity. After I explained to her that I was physically feeling terrible, she proceeded to tell me that I should pray. I did not take her seriously at first. I laughingly told her that although I thought prayer could be helpful to one's soul, it was not doing anything for my distended abdomen and could she please call the doctor to ask him if there was anything that could be done for me. The nurse, undaunted, told me that if I would only pray to Jesus Christ, I would feel better and that I did not need to talk to the doctor.

"All you have to do is say that you believe in Jesus as your savior and you will be fine."

I told her I was Jewish and I believed differently than she did, so would she call the doctor now. No, she insisted, she wanted to hear me pray first. At that point, I got very angry and told her that this was neither the time nor place for proselytizing and that I resented what she was trying to do. Finally, after a few more angry words she agreed to call the doctor and behaved rather hostilely towards me after that. When the doctor finally came, I whispered to him when the nurse left the room that she was trying to convert me but he did not believe me and did nothing. It turned out that it was necessary to insert a naso-gastric tube to relieve the painful pressure in my stomach. I was nervous about having the evangelizing nurse near me, but she was the only one there to help. She treated me very unkindly, jostling me about in a rough manner which, given my condition, was quite painful. Having a tube pushed up your nose and down your throat is one of the most awful procedures to endure. It is quite uncomfortable at best and excruciating at worst. The horror of being mistreated by and afraid of the nurse taking care of me was exceeded only by my fury at her religious presumptuousness. The next day I reported her to the patient relations department and requested that she stay away from me.

During my hospital stay, I was visited by Rabbi Levi Meier, the chaplain at Cedars. I remember having a very short conversation with him which ended with my asking for a prayerbook and Bible. In all honesty, I asked him for them because having a Rabbi in my room made me feel terribly guilty for what I was feeling about God. I thought if I really told him what I felt he would think I was a terrible person, certainly an awful Jew, and would not want to have anything to do with me. So I asked him for the prayerbook just to be polite, and he graciously obliged, bringing them up that very afternoon.

I have gone through many different phases in my religious observance. In recent years, I had become very attached to reading the Torah portion of the week every *Shabbat* and praying with the *minyan* (prayer group) that I had become a part of. It was a meaningful, religious act for me. While concentrating on a particular prayer or passage I would often feel connected to God, my heritage and deep parts of myself that were not touched by other means. I would always find something that spoke to my current concerns and feelings. But now, the mere thought of opening the books made me nauseous, and then I felt even more guilt for feeling that way. There were among my friends and acquaintances those who tried to "comfort" me in my time of illness with religious platitudes and stories which not only did I find distinctly unhelpful but, in fact, strongly resented.

A few days later, I decided that I needed some outlet for my thoughts or I was going to go crazy. One of my cousins had brought me a notebook and a pen, and I started to write a few of my thoughts down. Coincidentally, Rabbi Meier walked into the room as I was doing this. He greeted me, I said hello back, and then there was this awkward silence. I did not know what to say to him next. There was so much I needed to talk to someone about but did not know how to even start, so I handed him the notebook and shared what I had written. I had not written very much, just a few lines about my doubt and my anger. I wrote also about how I identified with our forefather, Jacob, who goes off and alone must wrestle through the night with a dark and shadowy assailant. I, too, felt that I was alone battling physical and emotional assailants. I was overwhelmed with what seemed like a perpetual struggle with an uncertain outcome. Rabbi Meier directed my attention to the end of that biblical interlude where Jacob, in overcoming his opponent, receives a special blessing, a new name, and so passes into a new state of being. He transcended his old reality to become something stronger and more aware than he was before through his painful struggle. This understanding helped me to focus on the dawn that would follow this dark ordeal. I found comfort in thinking that I would emerge from it all a stronger individual and that, perhaps, I would be able to find meaning in my experience.

There were different emotional phases I went through during my recovery and later, my convalescence. My focus initially was totally on "why me?" Later, it slipped into "why anyone?" and eventually enlarged to include the rest of the world's problems. This change of perspective is illustrated by my reactions to events that happened around me at the time. For example, I was watching a film one evening entitled "Whose Life Is It Anyway?," starring Richard Dreyfuss as an artist who becomes a quadriplegic as a result of a tragic accident. The movie is about his struggle to be allowed to die because he feels his life as it is now is meaningless. I knew what the film was about because I had seen the play some years before. In fact, I had designed the costumes for a college production of it, and I was curious to see how the movie version of the play was. It is an intense play but I did not expect my reactions to the issues involved to hit me as hard as they did. I found myself torn between compassion for this man whose life has been irrevocably changed, and fury with his decision to end it. My thinking went something like this: "How dare he decide to die when I am struggling so hard to survive. Why don't you learn to cope as I am? If he cannot make it, what makes me think I can?" I could not bear seeing someone else give up, especially someone bright, articulate and artistic. It came too close to my own feelings of despair and loneliness, too close to my insecurities. I make no claim of logic in any of my thoughts, but they made sense to me at the time. I began to realize that there were others in the world who were suffering, not just me. The better I got, the more I could see outside myself.

The next event of major significance was the massacre of Jews in an Istanbul synagogue by terrorists on September 6, 1986. My reaction to that was also very intense. The following is what I wrote in my journal the very next day:

It's 7:00 A.M., been up many hours this night. I am so sickened by yesterday's incident I can hardly stand it, and yet I must. What keeps running through my mind is on so many different levels of horror I hardly know which to start with, or for that matter whether I should start at all. There is a compulsion for me to express, to write, not to hide and scream at God inside myself. I can hardly see what I am writing because of the tears in my eyes that keep blinking themselves there despite my efforts to keep them in.

Shabbat yesterday went from Rosh Hashanah to Tisha B'Av (a Jewish Fast Day) to Yom Kippur in one day. It must have been that way for many people. Barbara (my aunt) called me after Shabbat to tell me what had happened so I would not see it first on the T.V. with the press's graphic footage. I did not need to see what happened; I knew what it would look like. Later, while I was watching something mindless on television, a news flash came on about Istanbul and I saw it all. My mind's image was pretty close to the reality.

So, what to do but go to sleep; there was no energy left in me to do much else. My grandmother, whom I talked to earlier, had obviously seen the news, too. I could hear it in the timbre of her voice as she tried to be cheerful on the phone. I can always hear the subtle changes in her voice when she is hiding something. I am worried about my father who is home alone since my mother is here in L.A. What demons will haunt his mind when he hears about this?

So, that is one layer of thoughts. Then all of my "why me?"'s of the past few days turned into "why us?," which has so many answers depending on your point of view as to be equally unanswerable. I do not even want to attempt to reconstruct my internal wanderings over that. Too big a matter and my mind kept leaping anyway. Twenty-two people. All saying the morning prayers. I kept thinking of the first line of the *Haftorah* (Isaiah 51:12): "I, even I, am He that comforts you; who are you, that you are afraid of man that shall die, and of the son of man that shall be made as grass." Somehow it is hard not to fear mankind who kill and the sons of men who though they may eventually wither as grass burn your bodies with gasoline first in the name of stupidity.

This morning started out so nicely. I read through the morning prayers for the first time since I got sick and all sorts of things jumped out at me from the text, especially any line that talked about hearts or death. It seemed so new and yet familiar, like meeting an old friend not seen in years. There was a sense of starting again, starting fresh, Rosh Hashanah-like, moments of looking inward and then the drive to look onward and ahead.

Then, in the evening, after the fateful phone call, I felt as if it were *Tisha B'Av*, as I mourned over the the deaths in my larger "family," furious at the senselessness of it all. The *Haftorah* (Prophets) that this morning seemed in many ways addressed to me personally, being one who has not yet gone "dying into the pit" and who has also "drunk much bitterness" recently, suddenly seemed kind of unhelpful and stale when applied to the larger scale of the world.

Once I got past thinking about that, I kept hearing the *Unesaneh Tokef* (an awe-inspiring prayer on the High Holidays) running through my head, and thoughts of the judgment of the year stopped my mental wanderings cold. Instead of thinking "Why was I being put through all this?," I began to think "Why did I survive all this?" Why were those people massacred? What have I done that allowed me life or what must I do to deserve the gift? I wonder, also, whether I have a long-term or a short-term loan. One never knows what will happen in the next moment, so you had better make this one worthwhile.

The final phase of all my thoughts, and there were many more I do not recall, was hearing the Martyrology from Yom Kippur in my head and mentally adding the Istanbul victims to the list. When I finally fell asleep, I dreamt that all the martyrs were spinning on the edge of a fiery cliff wrapped in bloody, burning prayer shawls and I could hear the tune of *Unesaneh Tokef* being sung. It was eerie. I wrote a poem about it.

Istanbul
On grey cliffs of martyrs memory
Where holy tempests swirl
In circled cycles
Trapped in furious spinning,
Flames leap up mountainsides,
Hungry for more kindling.
And quiet whispers of "Who shall live and who shall die"
Hiss below and above as
Bloody judgment falls
Silent as night.
And hollow voices echo, sighing,
Who will be remembered, who forgotten?
Who will say our names in echoing hallways?
Once a year, once a year,
When Akiba walks the shadowy list
Past lips and hearts to silent conclusion,

New figures will silhouette the page
To spin on grey and burning cliffs.

Convalescence

Being discharged from the hospital was wonderful and terrible at the same time. The thought of being home in my own apartment, in my own bed thrilled me. I could not wait to sleep a night through and not be bothered in the morning by some medical vampire who wanted to draw more blood. I wanted to reclaim my independence, do everything on my own and pick up my life right where I had left it, pretend that the last few months had never happened. Impossible dreamer, I.

Some people have the mistaken notion that getting out of the hospital means that you are all better and that everything is as it was. Not so. I completely underestimated how much life energy was necessary to initiate and complete even the basic tasks of living. In the hospital so much was done for me, meals prepared, bed linen changed, gowns washed, and there was always someone nearby if you needed help. Suddenly, I was on my own and even lifting a frying pan was a major undertaking. My father took off from work and came to Los Angeles to help me with the transition from hospital to my apartment which would have been nearly impossible without his help. For the next couple of weeks my grandmother cooked for me until I was strong enough to do simple food preparation on my own. I must note also that she brought me food when I was in the hospital, and I am convinced that her chicken soup contributed as much to my recovery as all the antibiotics.

I was alone most of the time during those long, recuperative months. My friends had returned to school and had little time for me. My roommate was also a busy student and I rarely saw her. It was several months before I felt strong and alert enough to drive, so I was basically homebound. I learned quickly which people really cared enough about me to visit or call. The first month after leaving the hospital my telephone was my lifeline. I needed to tell everyone I ever cared about that I was still here; I wanted them to know I was alive and thinking about them. I ran up a huge phone bill talking to friends I had not seen in a while. I was not at all sure how long I was going to live so I wanted to say hello and maybe goodbye to all those who mattered to me.

In general, my friends were sympathetic to me but they really did not understand how this experience had changed me. They were all healthy, active people under the age of thirty; none of them had anything nearly this catastrophic happen to them. This experience set me apart and alone from my peer group and contributed greatly to my post-surgery depression.

As time passed, I began to allow myself to acknowledge my anger and other feelings about what had happened to me. I found that just below the surface of the new pains and doubts lay all sorts of old emotional issues that I had never dealt with. The trauma of nearly dying and major surgery brought everything bubbling to the surface of my psyche. Anything bad that had ever happened to me was remembered; I mulled over old resentments, jealousies, abuses, misunderstandings. It appeared that I had to clear away all the old cobwebs and confront those events in my life that had made me so unhappy before I could move on to a brighter state of mind. It took me a long time to do that. I had to find a way to live with the constant awareness of death and the fear of illness. I had to learn how to cope with all the uncertainties of living and never really feeling safe or secure even with my own body. I had to learn how to "live" again. It did not come as easily as I or anybody who knew me expected it to.

The emotional and psychological affect of my heart surgery is still present to this day. It shows up in my attitudes, my goals, my conversations and my dreams. I have not been able to put it behind me and forget it because it is ever-present, from the internal ticking that I will hear for the rest of my life to the more unseen effects that dwell within my thoughts and emotions.

I view all events since that time through the filter of my heart surgery and near-death experience. I cannot help it; that is just the way it is. There are times when the perspective on life that experience gave me makes it much more meaningful to me and other times when I wish I could forget the whole thing. The following is an excerpt from a letter written to Rabbi Meier over a year after my surgery, describing some of my feelings during Rosh Hashanah and a dream which clearly reflected some of my thoughts and fears about death.

Davening (praying) this Rosh Hashanah was so intense, especially during the *Amidah* (central prayer). I found myself tuning out the words in front of me, or rather, my eyes got kind of blurry so I had to close them. I became almost hypnotized by the sound of my heart. Its constant tick was mantra-like and I felt my breath synchronizing with it, being conscious of each breath and hearing nothing but the sound of my breath and my heart. There ought to have been other noise, people noise--turning pages, coughing, whispers...but I heard nothing. It was as if I was in a vacuum.

I have never been much of a swayer when it comes to praying. In the religious high school I attended as a teenager, it was a sign of how devout you were and how "well" you prayed. The more active a *shuckler* (swayer) one was, the more religious. I hated this concept and subtly distinguished myself by never moving at all. I would find myself a quiet corner, preferably where I would not call attention to myself, and rigidly root myself to the spot. But this time as I stood totally immersed in my heartsound and my breathing, I became aware of my body moving back and forth just a little in the same rhythm. I felt as if I were gently floating in the air and being rocked almost imperceptibly by an invisible hand. I felt that my heartbeat and my life itself was a prayer.

The whole thing was so strange and so lovely. I felt infused with this strange unique warmth that I have only felt two other times in my life. It is so hard to write all this down; talking about this feels more difficult and personal than talking about one's love life. Putting words to experiences that defy words is to dilute them, yet I feel this urge to tell you about them, wanting to share just a little with someone I trust.

The first time, I experienced that strange warmth when I had the cardiac arrests in the hospital last year. I felt like I was floating then, too, except then it was in complete silence. I could not hear my heartbeat or my breathing since both had stopped. I experienced that same feeling again in a dream I had last night.

I dreamt I was getting married but I did not know to whom. I found myself walking up an aisle. There were people on either side of the aisle but I could not see who they were because I was looking straight ahead. I was wearing a white dress and had wildflowers in my hair. I felt luxuriously beautiful. I noticed that I was not wearing a veil and noted to myself that that was a good thing because I could see more clearly.

I walked up to the canopy and discovered that you and Rabbi Chaim Seidler-Feller were officiating. I turned around to see if my bridegroom was following me down the aisle. What I saw was not a human being but an essence of pure light. It was no color and all color at the same time, like a white hot flame floating towards me. This light-being settled itself next to me and as I turned towards it in wonder it wrapped itself like a ring around my finger. I lifted up my hand to look at it and suddenly it was all around me, or rather I was in the midst of it. I felt that strange, wonderful warmth all around me and inside me as if I were glowing from without and within.

I looked down and my wedding dress had turned into a *kittel* (a traditional Jewish burial garment) and my hair was all matted down as if someone had poured a pail of water on me from above. I heard my name and turned around to see who was calling me. In the aisle was a casket with the lid open, with six men in black standing next to it. I knew it was for me.

I turned back around to see if you were there and said something to the effect that I thought you were here to conduct my wedding, not my funeral. I fell weeping to the ground and said, "Levi, I wanted to be a blessing. Tell me I was a blessing. I wanted to be a prayer on someone's lips. I wanted to flow free like the water in my name. Tell me, was I?" You said you could not tell me but that the answer was in the casket. Still weeping I got up and lay down in the casket. The men put the lid on top. It was so dark and all I could hear was my heart ticking away. Then I woke up with a start.

The next morning I was thinking about the dream, and I remembered that in the readings from Erwin Altman's thoughts at your conference, he had written something about being a blessing that had struck such a powerful chord in me. There was a part about the individual connecting and uniting the wholeness of the self and the universe, as well as something about the word VEHEYEH (the Hebrew word for "and be") having the same letters as God's Name,

and what that meant about one's relationship to God. Anyway, that
was what this dream reminded me of.

My Rosh Hashanah prayer experience reflected the transformation of
my ticking heart valve from a constantly distressing annoyance into an
instrument for a spiritual experience. It was a sign of healing and the
meaningful integration of the near-death experience with my life. I shall
leave the analysis of my dream to those more qualified to do that, but say
only that its images are clearly related to issues from my heart surgery that
touched me deeply. It raised questions about the meaning and purpose of
my life, how I wanted to live and die.

I had attended the Psychology and Judaism Conference at
Cedars-Sinai where excerpts from Erwin Altman's "Reflections on this
Thing and No-Thing Called Life and Death" were read. "Reflections" was
a compilation of *Morenu* (our revered teacher) Altman's thoughts written
shortly before his death in 1986. The thoughts and philosophy expressed in
that paper (*Journal of Psychology and Judaism,* vol. 11, no. 2, Summer
1987) had a significant impact on me both consciously and, as is evident
from my dream, unconsciously as well. His personal life-philosophy was
drawn from the Divine Calling of God to Abraham, in which God directs
Abraham, "And Be a Blessing" -- *Veheyeh Berakhah* (Genesis 12:2). Being
a blessing had deep significance on many dimensions, including thought,
word and action. Being a blessing to *Morenu* Altman meant putting
"emphasis on man's actualization of his destiny within history, in the 'here
and now'... to use his comprehension to be and to become more and more
'A Blessing,' for the 'Wholeness' of himself and of all the creations of the
universe" (pp.122-23). As I struggled to find new ways of thinking about
my life, grappling with both existential and spiritual crises, Altman's motto
and thoughts offered a positive foundation for the beginning of the spiritual
and psychological healing process.

In her famous book, *On Death and Dying,* Elisabeth Kübler-Ross
describes five stages that a person with a terminal diagnosis may go
through: denial and isolation, anger, bargaining, depression and finally,
acceptance. When a catastrophic illness like the one that struck me occurs,
there is no time for that sequence of stages to develop. What I see in
retrospect is that I went through all those stages in one form or another after
I survived. It seemed to work for me in reverse, these being the steps I

needed to travel before being able to reenter life fully. My psyche was backtracking and taking the time it needed to get used to the death that almost happened, for which there was no time to prepare.

Have I reached acceptance yet? On some levels, yes and on some, no. There was a grieving that had to happen before I could be whole again. My heart had to mourn the loss not only of a valve, but of the sense of youthful invulnerability, the betrayal of the old God images it harbored and irrevocable changes in my physical and emotional being. This is growing pain of the highest order. I have yet to completely heal my heart, but I feel hopeful that each day's experience of life and love brings me closer to so doing.

CHAPTER 2

GROWING SICK:

THOUGHTS ON MONTHS AS A HEART PATIENT,

YEARS AS A RABBI

Rabbi William Cutter, Ph.D.

Pulitzer Prize-winner Annie Dillard (1989) once charged all would-be writers with a curious demand: "What would you begin writing if you knew you would die soon? What could you say to a dying person that would not enrage by its triviality?" If writing and reading about anything can be spoken of in such ultimate terms, how much more important must writing be when the very subject of the writing is death and illness itself!

There is a lot of writing about this subject, and many people buy books about illness. Each generation in America produces more literature about the subject: more stories, more hope of miraculous cure, more criticism of current medical practice, and more new language to do all that work. Metaphors abound to help us in the work of writing and reading, and the words used to describe our sickness and our health are especially rich and plentiful. The most interesting example of this linguistic excitement may be Jonathan Miller's *The Body in Question* (1978), in which the British physician-dramatist explains the very functions of our organs in terms of machinery from the industrial revolution. But the point is that language helps as we struggle to explain why being sick is so important.

Even universities tell young scholars that they will either publish or they will perish, which is really figurative language for announcing the importance of putting things into writing. The universities are right in another figurative way, and so I often suggest that patients keep a diary, some kind of record, of their experiences with serious illness.

Patients who write about their illnesses or who at least find the proper figures of speech to describe them have a way of gaining control, and a way of giving some concrete figuration to the potential emptiness that lies behind every illness. One either finds a way to deal with the emptiness, or one perishes to some extent.

My essay will have a lot to do with the metaphors of illness; and it will take advantage of some of that great abundance of writing that has been done over these past twenty years. Annie Dillard's words are appropriate for me in a surprising way: it was my own experience of illness and my own interest in writing about that illness that changed my thoughts about the meaning of illness and death. On the one hand, I learned that I had more spiritual layers -- higher levels of consciousness, if you will; and on the other hand, I learned to pay more attention to my immediate and very physical surroundings, so I learned also to touch "lower" more everyday realities. I learned to keep my inner eye on thoughts about God's purposes, while (in Milton Steinberg's words), embracing the physical world with open arms. And I learned about some often neglected issues in medical care.

The drama of illness made me more interested in living, in general. My interest began with my first moments in the hospital when I recalled Paddy Chayevsky's movie "Hospital" and worried that my urine test was going to be confused with someone else's; and it continues eleven years later, when I hear the stories that sick people tell me as I visit with them and their families. Although I felt quite ill, I was able to pay close attention to all kinds of things within the hospital: pictures on the wall, the way elevators felt as I was being wheeled around, the atmosphere of x-ray rooms, the sounds of people's voices and the reassurances of kind doctors. I have not lost my acuity for detail. Even my fantasies seem to have been permanently nourished, from my early experience with semi-consciousness. I once figured out, for example, that the monitors which were hooked up to record my heartbeat were actually keeping me alive. And in the intensive care unit I dreamed about a desert island and idyllic tropical settings during a brief episode of shock from a potassium deficiency. At the time I wondered why the name of that island was "Ischemia," and only later did I realize that ischemia is the name for lack of blood and oxygen in the coronary arteries. I still remember the sounds in the darkening life I was to inherit; and although the acoustics of memory have distorted some, they have provided a link between what I experienced and what I now believe.

Perhaps a rabbi should talk about what he believes. On my last day in the hospital, after seven months of admissions and releases, Rabbi Meier, the hospital chaplain, asked me how all of this experience had affected my belief in God. No one had ever asked that question of this rabbi before. The question was the first step in insinuating a religious frame of reference into my life, and a commitment to activity in and around health and disease: working with sick people, and helping my own students think more about the place of illness and wellness in their own training to minister to people's needs. To my surprise, the experience has helped me combine my more purely academic work with the real lived experience of people. I teach literature, and living life a little closer to the edge made me a better reader.

All those little things I had begun to notice during my first hours in the hospital were suddenly a composite of a much bigger and more meaningful universe. God is, indeed, in the details.

It is, then, a gift for some of us to have been sick. In the perfect world toward which Jewish tradition points, but which no tradition really believes has come, perhaps no one would be ill. But in the imperfect world we inhabit, it is sometimes necessary to experience wellness and illness as part of one continuum. If for me as a rabbi, the notion of having to die before one can live is incomprehensible, at least I can say that one may have to be sick in order to appreciate being well. I am, in general, grateful for the experience, if not always for the inconveniences I now live with. And I may qualify, by pure accident, for something that Professor Lewis Thomas would like to expect from his medical students: urging that all future doctors be made to undergo one serious viral illness in their early professional careers so that they would know what it is like to be sick.

Thomas has been worried over the years that doctors are increasingly estranged from their patients' feelings. Tracing this tendency to the time when the stethoscope replaced the doctor's ear against the patient's chest, Thomas (1983) has been able to accept the realities of technology while warning of its spiritual costs. I learned that all professions have their versions of being far away from their clients' heartbeats. And that has religious meaning as well.

I have hesitated to write about my medical experiences for public purposes. There is no false humility here, just a wondering if a healthy person ought to go around announcing his good fortune. I do not usually exhibit my cardiac scars around the hospital, for example, but when it seems appropriate, I do tell patients that I have been through serious cardiac surgery in order to encourage them to be optimistic. Now I can enjoy the twist of phrase that I sometimes publicize because I did not perish. So perhaps this is another legitimate instance of sharing my scars. How was my experience like that of everyone else? What might they learn from what happened to me?

What happened to me is similar to what happens to anyone who becomes sick suddenly. One day you are well, and the next day you are sick, and you cannot even be certain where the dividing line between the two conditions was laid down. Fortunately most of us who become sick develop a kind of amnesia which eradicates fear about being sick again, or about re-experiencing the initial dark panic. But, of course, I do remember the moment when my illness became apparent. And I remember the awkward choreography between my wife, who was on the phone at the time, and me as I was trying to gain access to the line. (We have since put in other lines.) It was a deeply personal and maritally telling moment in our lives, but probably no different from the story of any other person who seems to get sick all of a sudden. As the great *Village Voice* writer, Paul Cowan, said of his own illness (1988): "We are all going to enter the land of the sick at one time in our lives. The question is only when."

On that evening over ten years ago, in order to determine which land of the sick I was entering, the young doctor at Cedars-Sinai Medical Center greeted me at the door to the emergency room. "What are you feeling?," he asked. "Is it like an elephant sitting on your chest?" And before slipping off into my ischemic fantasies, I found enough sarcastic energy to tell him that I had never had an elephant sitting on my chest. Although his question was innocent enough, it has always served as a reminder to me of two important truths about the sensitivity of patients. First, I learned that the people who are devoted to patients' health really must communicate carefully, since patients are especially sensitive. Second, I learned that because patients are so sensitive, it is nearly impossible to avoid saying something that might offend them. This realization has given me the strength to go into hospital rooms, to serve as a chaplain and to return to a kind of religious life to which I had originally intended to devote myself. In order to be able to help people you have to intuit their emotions, and thus reduce the risk of damaging their faith in you; but in order to begin the process, you have to be willing to take risks. I suspect that some rabbis do not visit patients enough because they are afraid of doing something ineffectual.

I learned something else from having started my journey in the emergency room. I call it the paradox of self-help. One of the most important things patients can do for themselves is to take responsibility for understanding their illnesses and for their own medical management. The "mode" of relationship with a physician has to be one of mutual respect and interdependence.

But those who enter the hospital in a state of emergency begin in just the contrary mode: one of total dependence, weakness and gratitude for the strength of doctors and nurses. Most acutely ill patients have little capability of worrying about the development of mutual relationships with those who are helping.

Because I was lying on my back for the first several days in cardiac care units, I felt especially helpless. Every paternal or maternal reassurance by others and every kind and supportive word was encoded in my memory bank. It was some trick learning that this would not be an appropriate attitude for taking care of myself over the long haul. It took many years to move towards autonomy, but it is a move we all must make.

So if you ask me what I have learned from my illness, the answer would have to do with understanding the very particularity of life; its concreteness and actuality. I learned about loss of power and about gaining it back; I learned some subtleties of interpretation; and I learned how to use memory for creative purposes. In my awareness of that sense of the real and the immediate, and the very tangible aspects of living, I have moved away from what had been a latent interest in traditional medical ethics questions and into a greater concentration on the day-to-day needs of patients. Along with Rabbi Levi Meier, I have come to call this area "soft ethics." This division of ethical studies has some parallels in the Jewish tradition's distinction between legal behavior (known as *halacha*), and more nuanced spiritual values (known as *musar* or *aggadah*).

The aspects of medical ethics which fascinate me now concern how patients experience their illnesses in the day-to-day business of being ill. While the more dramatic questions of life and death, medical experiments, transplants, euthanasia and abortion continue to be the stuff of which conferences are composed, for most patients and for most doctors there is a long agenda of items that fill the ill patient's day.

For every medical question about when life ends, and whether a patient is entitled to die at will, there are a hundred questions with ambiguous answers in which doctor and patient have to negotiate the daily terrain. How, for example, can a very sick patient be made to feel better about the cost of services? How might a nurse or front office manager create a hospitable frame within which the patient is treated? How much time can a doctor legitimately afford to spend with a patient, given the realities of overhead, reluctant insurance companies, and the pressure on the doctor from family and community? What can a patient's friends and associates do to ensure that the patient does not feel abandoned by the community? What are the things one might say to make a person feel stronger and more in charge of the future? How can a doctor relieve a patient of the burden of a nagging spouse? Where do nurses fit into a doctor's plan? And, finally, how can all of us help to get our language clear so that we more or less know what the other person is saying? Are there metaphors more suitable to ethical relationships?

For the most part, I find Jewish bioethics "out of sync" with the real and desperate needs of people, and not related to the most pressing areas in which Jewish life impinges on the medical situation: doctors' fees; the personal suffering of the families of ill people, and the abrasive interaction between family members; the dignity of patients who are suffering the indignity of illness; the chaotic way in which families of ill people have to make decisions; and the loneliness of all the people going through the tunnel of illness. For my students who will lead communities some day, there are problems on a larger scale which will involve them in building facilities: what can we do about hospital architecture to make patients and their families feel more human? Are there places to sit down when talking with a doctor? Do the walls of testing rooms look like prison cells or do they look like helping environments? What does it feel like to spend your illness looking up at people's nostrils? How, in general, can communities come to understand that the care of people in trouble is an ethical priority, inspiring us to make it possible to be ill and to feel human at the same time?

David Hartman has called some of these problems the "moral uncertainties" in the practice of medicine (1979); and attending to them has been called "redeeming the intangible" in medical practice (De Vries, 1979). As David Hartman has said: "Good medical practice requires knowledge which depends, in part, on the existence of relationships of trust and the absence of embarrassing dependency." I know few physicians who would disagree with this statement; but I know few who do anything about it. Thus, as another Jewish scholar, Aaron Lichtenstein, has insisted (1975), there are two moralities: a morality of duty (the traditional legalistic side of the ledger), and the morality of aspiration (the softer ethics).

The contemplation of specific solutions to specific problems can enrich our ethical perspectives; and the traditional scholars of medical ethics have contributed enormously to our understanding of the meeting place of technology and religious values. But if the more traditional ethical questions are allowed to control the agenda, we shall surely use these problems to divert us from the intangible and persistent problems with which all patients live even when traditional moral questions are not at stake. But I am not certain that this message can be compelling to people who have not been ill themselves.

One curious result of my experience has been an interest in the profession of medical doctor. In this profession I have seen a kind of model for "profession" or professionalism. I share this idea with the Protestant theologian Stanley Haurwas (1977), who has suggested that doctors may represent a useful body of people in whom to anchor our interest in professional identity, and about whom to ask all kinds of questions about what a profession is. I am a rabbi, for example, but through my awkward and wonderful experiences with doctors, I was often able to gain an insight into my own behavior and the behavior of my colleagues. I am still not certain which viruses should be injected into our seminary classrooms, but I am certain that we understand the wrong things about our clients. And I have found Haurwas a convincing entry point to this kind of thinking, from which ultimately all particular experience can be universalized.

The medical relationship, i.e., the connection between the doctor and the patient, captures the tragedy of the human condition. Nowhere else do we feel as impotent to reach perfection, to achieve satisfaction, or to address social problems on a broad basis. Every human relationship reflects human limits in one way or another, but because of the possible life and death implications of this relationship, medicine is a paradigm for those limits. Annie Dillard would like this thought. And Haurwas insists that medicine is an important area for moral reflection because there we have raised with particular cogency questions no moral person can avoid. Thus medicine can be an important form of human activity that helps us to chart our way in other aspects of our lives. Thinking such as this stands behind us when we take the questions addressed to doctors and ask them of ourselves. In a slightly paradoxical way, it is the existence of this very technical and hard scientific profession that makes us understand the unity of humanity; the similarity between the problems in the discourse of science and the intangible aspects of our lives; and the continuity between wellness and illness.

Learning about these connections has helped me be a better rabbi, I think; but it has also helped me understand the place of hard science in a life where I might be tempted (as a defensive maneuver, I now see) to reject hard science in the interest of what I used to call "higher things." The world can best be understood as a sum of integrated parts, for even ethics and hopes are linked; and problems are systems made up of resolutions and new problems. Both hard science and soft science people, as well as rigorous ethical theorists and soft ethicists, need to get along better.

My own hope is that we will judge human behavior increasingly in terms of aspiration instead of right or wrong; I hope that legalistic norms may be informed by spiritual frameworks in which scholars like Lichtenstein, Hartman, Thomas and Haurwas work. For the scientific sometimes beckons even the humanists to use ethics to hide from the compromising problems which face us every day. The questions of bioethics are important, to be sure, just as scientific medicine will have a lot to do with making people feel well. But the bigger questions we must help professionals confront is in what kind of medical world are they going to be practicing their bioethics and their medical science?

These reflections have made me serve people more expansively and have placed my own experience with illness in a framework where new meanings have emerged within my life. I am not a physician, but I am a kind of healer, just as physicians represent a kind of priestly function. I am thankful for these insights, and I hope that more and more people will be able to come to some of them without the "benefit" of the risky business of being sick. Death may be easier to deal with than illness in some instances. At least it is accompanied by prescriptions. It is clear cut, with more refined definition. Illness often involves us in hurt feelings and complicated relationships which endure throughout our lives. But the point is that death and life are related, and one of the connecting tissues is illness itself.

I will end with an anecdote that may illustrate the connection between death and life, and certainly illustrates the discomfort which many have with that connection. I was seated with my students in the lobby of our largest hospital a few years ago, when a local surgeon stopped to visit. He was surprised to see me there, and he asked whether someone had died. Someone was indeed dying, but we were visiting that patient and others who were on our visiting list for that day. The surgeon rather liked the idea of training rabbis to visit sick people and their families. He knew that rabbis often visited, but he had not thought of it in terms of any specific training that might be carried on in a training program. Not, at least, until he had asked the question: "What are you doing here? Has someone died?"

A few days later one of the patients did indeed die; and I received a phone call during a faculty meeting at our school. My colleagues on our school faculty know of my work at the hospital; they see it as a training opportunity for our students to visit sick people, and we had discussed the course briefly at this very meeting. The call that interrupted us was from one of our local mortuaries, whose director was calling at the request of the patient's wife who wanted me to conduct the funeral. A secretary interrupted our meeting and said aloud that the mortician requested that I come "right over!" One of my faculty colleagues, more used to my activities in visiting patients in my academic role, looked up from his notes and asked: "What is the matter? Is someone sick?"

References

Cowan, Paul. (1988). In the land of the sick. *The Village Voice*, May 17.

De Vries, Marco. (1979). *The redemption of the intangible in medicine.* Rotterdam: Erasmus University.

Dillard, D. Annie. (1989). *The New York Times Book Review,* May 28.

Fox, Marvin, ed. (1975). Does Jewish tradition recognize ethics independent of halakha? In *Modern Jewish ethics.* Columbus: Ohio State University Press.

Hartman, David. (1975). Moral uncertainties in the practice of medicine. *The Journal of Medicine and Philosophy,* 4 (1).

Haurwas, Stanley. (1977). *Truthfulness and tragedy.* South Bend: University of Notre Dame Press.

Jakobovits, Immanuel. (1975). *Jewish medical ethics.* New York: Bloch.

Lamm, Maurice. (1972). *The Jewish way in death and mourning.* New York: Jonathan David.

Lichtenstein, Aaron. (1975). In *Modern Jewish ethics,* ed. by Marvin Fox. Columbus: Ohio State University Press.

McPhee, John. (1984). Heirs of general practice. *The New Yorker,* July 23.

Miller, Jonathan. (1981). *The body in question.* New York: Random.

Rosner, Fred et al. (1979). *Jewish bioethics.* New York: Hebrew Publishing Company.

Starr, Paul. (1984). *The social transformation of American medicine.* New York: Basic.

Thomas, Lewis. (1983). *The youngest science: Notes of a medicine watcher.*
New York: Viking.

CHAPTER 3

THE DOCTOR IN THE PATIENT:

THE PATIENT IN THE DOCTOR

Rabbi Harold M. Schulweis, Th.D.

Mama encapsulated an entire world of Jewish values into two Yiddish words. If a glass was broken or money lost, or property robbed, Mama would respond, *"Abi gezunt,"* as long as you have your health. And if I sneezed, which was frequent owing to my allergic reaction to cats, dust and pollen, Mama would rush in and with her hand pull both of my ears upwards while crying out, *"Gezuntheit."* Years later when I observed the misshapen ears of *Star Trek*'s clever Mr. Spock, I concluded (a) that Spock must have suffered from allergy, and (b) that he must have been repeatedly blessed by a Jewish mother.

The Primacy of Health

The primacy of health which entered the ethos of the family is rooted in the passionate Jewish affirmation of life. No matter the wretchedness of the human condition, life remains holy. And so the folk tale of Reb Moshe, a poor man gathering sticks of wood in the forest, placing them in a torn sack, throwing it over his bony shoulders and then stumbling. The sticks scatter to the earth and Reb Moshe cries out, *"Ribbono Shel Olam* - Master of the Universe - send the Angel of Death and take me from this earth." As if in response to his prayer, the Angel of Death appears out of nowhere. "You called for me, Reb Moshe?"   "Yes, yes," Reb Moshe stammers. "Would you help me gather these sticks?"

However frustrating our lot, health and life are sacred. "For a one-day-old child who is ill, the Sabbath may be violated. For a King David deceased it may not be desecrated" (Talmud, *Shabbat* 151b). *"Hamira sakkanta meissura"* - violating one's health is a greater transgression than violating ritual. If health is sacred, the physician is endowed with a special measure of sanctity.

The Physician

In medieval times, the physician was called to the Torah by no less a title than *morenu* - our teacher. Jewish codes declared that a physician could pray his prayers before the statutory time so as to be free to visit his patients. The doctor could shorten the days of his own mourning to attend to his patients, even if other doctors were available, since patients respond best to their own doctors.

The doctor and the patient are bound by a mystique. Between them there is more than an exchange of goods and services. Between them is health and sickness, life and death. Healing depends upon their intimate relationship. The patient enters the doctor's office prepared to reveal the most personal secrets of his body and soul. He stands naked before the physician, exposing his private scars, blemishes, fears and anxieties. The doctor, in turn, has chosen to enter the gray world of complaints, screams and moans. It is no minor decision to assume the burdens of diagnosis and prognosis, to prescribe potent medicines and intrusive modalities. A medical misjudgment is not a grammatical mistake.   It may prove to be an incorrigible and even fatal decision.

The rabbis knew how filled with anxiety the doctor's decisions must be. In a section of the codes (*Yoreh De'ah* 336) they urged the physician not to despair. Let him not think, "Who needs the anguish of this practice? What if I err and cause the death of this patient?" They warned against the thinking which would lead the physician to argue, "God afflicts man with illness, shall I then interfere with His will and offer cures?" The rabbis interpreted Exodus 21:19, "He shall surely cause him to be healed," to counter the theology of human non-intervention. He who relieves suffering imitates the ways of the Faithful Physician. He who restrains his hand from healing the sick out of mistaken piety is deemed as one who sheds the blood of God's creation.

Ideally the doctor-patient relationship is a covenant of comradeship which shadows the covenant between God and the physician. But in fact, what has the patient in common with the physician? They each come from different stations and are endowed with different status. The doctor is healthy. He enters the hospital room dressed in a white, starched uniform, armed with charts and X-rays, EKG's, EEG's. He understands the undulating curves, the monitoring apparatus and the bizarre soundings of the mysterious beepings.

The Patient

Etymology points to the difference: *doctor*, teacher; *patient - patoir*, suffering.

The patient is sick, frightened and ignorant, hanging on to every inflection, to every intonation of the doctor's voice. They place bracelets with the patient's name upon his wrist as with a newborn baby. He is infantilized, protected by iron rails attached to a mechanized bed. He lies obedient to every order issued by any uniformed authority.

The patient may revert to infancy, not simply because the system forces his regression. He is tempted, despite his occasional demurrers, to surrender his autonomy. He endows his physician with miraculous powers. He would transform the stethoscope into a magic wand and the illegible prescription into an *elixir vitae*. The doctor is apotheosized, made into a savior, redeemer, god.

The Myth of Omnipotence

With the surrender of self, the healing relationship is jeopardized. For therapy is a synergistic action, a cooperative venture between the healer and he who seeks to be healed. For the sake of the therapy, the physician must guard against seduction by the patient. He must resist the heady intoxication of the sick man's flattery.   The patient would have him omnipotent, omniscient, ubiquitous.   Every patient wishes to believe that his physician is the brightest and the best.   Should he buy into the patient's adoration, the physician will be weighed down with unconscionable burdens. Should he prove fallible, or come late or himself grow sick, it will be taken as betrayal and unforgivable failure.   Should he stumble or falter, the physician who was lionized yesterday will be demonized tomorrow.

Flattered by the omnipotent wish of the infantilized patient, the doctor may well grow aloof.   His "coldness" stems less from conceit than from fear.   Cast by the patient in the armor of infallibility, he turns impassible. Who can live up to the mystique of invulnerability without distancing himself from the idolatrous patient?

The doctor may enjoy the myth of omnipotence, and the patient may find perverse comfort in self-induced paralysis.   The latter feels himself bathed in moral anesthesia.   "I am helpless.   I can do nothing.   You, doctor, cure, heal, operate, excise, exorcise."   The physician has lost the indispensable ally in the battle against disease.   The patient has lost the curative powers breathed into his nostrils by the source of life.   Will, hope, trust and the vitality of his recuperative energy are abandoned.   The healing is endangered, the relationship is injured.

Who knows where psyche ends and soma begins?   Who knows how the spirit addresses the body?   Jewish tradition is especially aware of the healing power of self-respect and the attitude of affirmation.   When Hezekiah, the King, fell ill, God spoke to the prophet Isaiah, "Son of Amoz, go and tell the King, 'Set your affairs in order, for you are going to die. You will not live.'"   Then Hezekiah, hearing Isaiah's message, rose and turned to the prophet.   "The way of the world is for a person who is visiting the sick to say, 'May heaven have mercy upon you.'   And the physician continues to tell him to eat this, to drink this and not that.   Even when the physician realizes that his patient approaches death, he does not say: 'Arrange your affairs,' lest the patient's mind grow faint."   This tradition of courage comes to us from King David.   "Even if a sharp sword is placed against the throat of man, let him not despair.   As Job declared, 'Though He slay me, yet will I trust'" (Ecclesiastes *Rabbah*; B.T. *Berakhot*).   In *articulo mortis*, in the teeth of death, the patient must not surrender to pitiless doom.

Hope is no vain gesture. "Hope must never die too far ahead of the patient."

What have they in common, the doctor and the patient? Most important, the healing and liberating knowledge that in every doctor there is a patient and that in every patient there is a doctor. The two comrades who struggle in common against pain and disease must release each other from the myths which tear the healing relationship apart. The patient must respect the doctor's competence and loyalty while acknowledging his fallibility and vulnerability. The physician must respect the patient's suffering while reminding him of his own strength and curative powers. Healing is a dialogue of trust between the two. The doctor and the patient have this in common: they are persons. Persons in covenant, aware of the wonder of each other's humanity, may heal.

CORONARY CONNECTIONS:

FROM A HOSPITAL,

SOME SECRETS OF THE HEART REVEALED

Rabbi Harold M. Schulweis, Th.D.

Some attribute the statement to Santayana, others to Einstein. "We cannot know who first discovered water, but we can be sure it was not the fish." Why not the fish? Because water is all about them; they breathe it, taste it, swim in it. For them, water is too obvious to be noticed. Could it be that only when they are caught in the fisherman's net, trembling, gasping for air, the revelation occurs to them?

Water is life. Water is our life.

We humans are born into life. It is in us, in our being. It pulsates in our veins. We sleep and rise up into life; and often we are late, sometimes too late, to discover it. In our infantile omnipotence, we take our immortality as given. To those who, like the fish, take their life support system for granted, the powerful biblical reminder - "therefore, choose life that you shall live" (Deuteronomy 30:19) is addressed.

When we are removed from the vital source of our energy, when we tremble, gasp for air, flail about wildly to grab at a straw of life, then it is that we catch a glimpse of the miracle of breathing, seeing, touching, hearing, smelling, feeling. In *extremis*, old sayings, cliched greetings - *"zei gezunt," "l'chayim"* - sound profound truths.

Surrounded by catheters and monitors and masks and needles, faced with the real possibility of my incapacitation and my death, I am jolted by transforming revelations. Fear and trembling are fierce instructors of the human spirit. "Do you not know that there comes a midnight hour when we must unmask? Do you suppose that life will forever suffer itself to be treated as a joke? Do you suppose that one can slip out a little before the midnight hour?" (Soren Kierkegaard)

"Every man is a child and pain is his teacher" (Alfred de Musset). Out of sickness and pain and fear, prayers once mechanically recited, benedictions mindlessly changed, take on a new pertinence.

"Make you a new heart and a new spirit, for why will you die?" (Ezekiel 18:31) I hear with new ears. I see with new eyes this prayer I have recited from my childhood: "Blessed art Thou who has formed the human being in wisdom and created in him a system of veins and arteries. It is well known before Thy glorious throne that if but one of these openings be closed, it would be impossible to exist in Thy presence." Once I thought this a primitive prayer - not of dreams or refined petitions - but of openings and closings, orifices, apertures, cavities of my own flesh. How unseemly a prayer, how lacking in aesthetics, how out of place within the covers of our majestic liturgy. But now I read it with new amazement and respect for its penetrating candor and concreteness.

Real prayer is with your body and your soul, with your bones and your flesh, and about your whole being. "The soul is Thine and the body is Thine. Blessed art Thou, O Lord, who healest all flesh and doest wonders."

Doest wonders. That is what prayer is about, to dissolve the boredom that dulls our senses, to open our eyes to the miracles that are daily with us - evening, morn, and noon. Prayer is not boring. We are boring. Prayer is the antidote to yawning. Prayer means to overcome the pedestrian perspective. Menachem Mendel of Kotzk chastised those who walk through life "with honey smeared on the soles of our shoes."

Pay attention. The sand beneath our sandals is holy. We walk on sacred soil, this amazing earth on which we tread.

I have been shaken by the shoulders of my being, awakened to life-and-death options. As one of T.S. Eliot's characters put it, "I have seen the moment of my greatness flicker, and I have seen the Eternal Footman hold my coat and snicker - and, in short, I was afraid."

But fear has its wisdom. Out of real fear, the fear of life and death, a thousand petty anxieties and dangers evaporate. Out of fear comes lucidity and out of lucidity a different understanding. When I have seen the shadow of death, and have lived to remember its face, how am I so readily frustrated with the myriad irritations, brooding over imperfections, failures, flaws?

"The Lord is my light and my healing; whom shall I fear? The Lord is the stronghold of my life; of whom shall I be afraid?" (Psalm 27)

Out of real fear, the glimpse of a new consciousness, a new gratitude is born.

Knowing mortality, what ambitions do I seek, what achievements, what acquisitions, what thrills, what childish fantasies of the rich and the famous? Why so full of complaints and demands? "I want, I want..."

Do you want what you want?

What do you crave with your insatiable neediness?

And where do you look for transcendence? Is there not wonder enough in your world? Will you forget the ecstasies of life, those post-operative marvels, the wonders, the signs, the miracles - to turn freely in your own bed from side to side, to cough, to sneeze, to walk, to wash without pain and fatigue?

Nissim, miracles - not in mountains moving or seas splitting, or people walking on the surface of waters - but in the rapture of breathing and sighing, in understanding a word spoken or a paragraph read, in following an argument, in recognizing a face, in waking to the ecstasy of ordinariness, the extraordinary ordinariness:

> "A solitary stroll through the streets; windows, tastes, colors, a dark climb-up the stairs, broken, crooked, a good *shabbos* greeting to uncle and aunt. Hallah dunked in red wine, pepper-sprinkled fish with white horseradish, green-red Sabbath fruit cherries, currants, gooseberries, the sourest of gooseberries between tart teeth." (Yaakov Glatstein)

I wonder at the restless searchers, the voyagers for spirituality, looking for mystic signs, special mantras, seances, levitations, transmigration, trance-channeling communications with the dead, flirtations with extra-terrestrials. Not that I am unmoved by the yearning for the transcendent, by the hunger for communion with another dimension beyond the flat surface of a material world that might offer this planet greater meaning. But they seek for God and wonder and spirituality in outlandish places, climbing the mountains, plumbing the depths of oceans.

Where else should they seek spirituality? Reb Eizek, son of Yekel of Cracow, dreamed that he was to look for a treasure beneath the bridge in Prague. He trusted the dream and set off to Prague. But the bridge was guarded by soldiers and he dared not dig. One day, the captain of the guard asked him what he was doing, standing day after day at the bridge. Reb Eizek told him he was following the mandates of a dream. "And so to please a dream you have traveled from Cracow to Prague. I too had a dream, that there is a treasure beneath the oven of a Jew in Cracow. The Jew's name was Eizek, son of Yekel." The captain laughed. Eizek bowed and returned to Cracow and dug up the treasure.

The treasure is not elsewhere. It is close to you, in your neighborhood, within your people, all about you.

It is not far off in the heavens above or the depths beneath, but in you. "In thy mouth and in thy heart."

Consider the heart, the soul of life. One half pound, the size of a closed fist, pumping blood through vessels more than one hundred thousand miles long, pumping blood ten thousand times a day. This heart, now wounded, scarred, occluded, atrophied, is deliberately stilled, the patient anaesthetized, marsupialized, heparinized, intubated, cannulated. The patient prepared, subject to hypothermia, cardioplegia, oxygen pumped to allow skillful courageous hands to sever sternum bone and muscle, to penetrate the heart itself so that it can be given life.

Who now dares take life for granted? Who can yawn in the face of this... worldly resurrection? Whose tongue can remain locked, whose lips sealed before such awesome wonder? Who cannot but offer benediction before the surgeon and his team and declare: "Blessed art Thou, O Lord our God, who shares His wisdom with flesh and blood."

Who can rant against science and technology, as if they stood in opposition to faith and religion? Are these marvelously contrived machines not instruments of divinity? Blessed is the human mind who can put together fragmented parts, make strong fragile organs, circumvent dead parts, and connect life with life. Look where for miracles? We carry them in our flesh and blood.

Blessed is the curative wisdom of the body.

We pray wrong. To pray is not to pay off your debt to some celestial creditor. It is not some unnatural act of piety. To pray is to notice, to pay attention, to overcome the apathy of entitlement. I look with new eyes at the opening prayers of our daily service, bursting with gratitude for opening the eyes to the blind, for raising up those bowed down, for guiding the step, for strengthening the weary.

I am not the only one who has been afflicted by illness, not the only one frightened by death and to life, but I now have a knowledge different from that drawn from texts. Knowledge by acquaintance is different from knowledge by description. It is one thing to read about it, or to hear about it from another, and something else to offer testimony out of your own flesh. I have come out of this, not with revelations, but with the testimony of old truths renewed.

For Judaism life is holy - not life in another time or another place, not life in heaven among angelic forms - but this one here and now with all its human agonies and frustrations. There is basic to Judaism an intense thirst for life.

Life is the major attribute of God - He is *chai ha-olamim,* life of the universe. To desire life is to desire God. To destroy life in oneself or another is to loathe God. We are bidden to fall in love with life again, to seize hold of this day and rejoice in its marvel.

The rabbinic tradition reminds us that laws and ordinances are for life, "that man shall live by them and not die by them" (Leviticus 18:5, *Sanhedrin* 74a). And in one of the major rabbinic codes we read that whoever asks whether or not it is permissible to desecrate the Sabbath in order to save life is "as if he sheds blood," (Jerusalem Talmud) and whichever scholar is asked that question is reprehensible because diligent religious teachers should have taught clearly so that the question would never have been raised.

Life is holy and life is plural - as it is grammatically plural in the Hebrew term *chayim.* What a conceit to think of myself as a self-sufficient biosystem, a portable set of plumbing, a self bounded by my outer skin. What a deceit is played upon us by the false intimacy of "me" or "I." There is no solitary life. There is no I without Thou, no "me" without "us." For our life, we are profoundly dependent upon each other.

The evidence stares me in the face. A call went out for blood contributions and was answered with quiet, anonymous dignity. But consider, in our biblical tradition, "blood is life." We are warned not to shed the other's blood, not to stand idly by the spilled blood of the victim and to spill the blood of the slaughtered animal upon the ground so as not to drink of its life. But you are not mandated to transfuse your blood into another's veins, to put your God-given vitality into another. What, then, does it mean voluntarily, out of care and concern and love, to share of your life with another, save to enact an imitation of God?

I stare at the intravenous vessel. Am I indeed a solitary, discrete, self-sufficient, independent creature? How foolishly tragic is Narcissus gazing at his own reflection. Your vitality courses through my veins. My energy is derived from yours. Can we ignore our interdependence? We need one another. We are each other's life - in sickness and in health.

In the Jewish prayer for healing we pray not "heal me, O Lord, and I will be healed," but "heal us, O Lord, and we shall be healed. Blessed art Thou, O Lord, who heals the sick of Thy people."

No postoperative praise of illness and suffering is intended. I do not mean that illness and pain are somehow good, that because they can sensitize us, fear and suffering are somehow justified. Sickness, pain, anguish, torment and death are neither rewards nor punishments from God. In our tradition, it is not piety, but blasphemy to pursue martyrdom for its own sake. But how and what we learn from adversity, how we raise private trauma into public morale is the way we add dignity to God's name. Not the suffering, but the refusal to let it subdue our will to live; not the pain, but the courage and hope that enable us to overcome despondency are the signs of God's goodness and reality. No one struck me down from above to punish me for my transgressions - God is no sadist. No one struck me down from above to reward me with new insight - God is no clumsy instructor. But God gave me mind and heart to learn divine matters from natural events.

I have learned that God's language is in human behavior; that we are God's alphabet from *aleph* to *tav*. We are God's vocabulary.

Consider the story based on the ambiguous biblical verse: "Charity averts death." Whose death? His mother is ill. The son quickly calls for an ambulance to take her to the hospital. In the midst of the turmoil his father whispers to him that it is Friday and that he should not forget to bring home a stranger for the Sabbath meal. The young man is disturbed that his father would think of poor strangers when his mother is in such dire straits.

But days later he says to his father: "Now I understand, father, about the stranger. You wanted to save Mother's life. 'Charity averts death.'" "No," says the father. "What I asked you to do I did not because I thought it would avert Mother's death, but because 'charity averts God's death.'"

Without charity, without love, God dies in this world. We are God's witnesses. If we are alive to each other, God is alive. If we live and love and help and heal, God is confirmed. God's name is exalted.

We prove God's goodness not by philosophic argument, but through the demonstration of our relationship with His world. In our behavior we argue God into existence on earth as He is in Heaven.

I have learned from this experience that friendship in family and in community is sacred, and that it is a foolish canard to declare that "words are cheap." A letter, a card, a prayer are life transfusions of the human spirit. A call or a visit is as therapeutic as the cleverest of medicines; our ancient sages did not exaggerate when they wrote, "He who visits the sick causes him to live" (*Nedarim*).

Do not diminish the *mitzvah* (commandment) of *bikkur cholim*, visiting the sick. There is an ethics, an aesthetics, an art in visiting the sick. In the *Shulchan Aruch (Yoreh De' ah* 335:4,5,8), the visitor is counselled to "speak with discretion and tact, so as neither to revive him (with false hopes) nor depress him (with words of despair); not to visit a patient whose condition is an embarrassment to him or for whom conversation is difficult."

Why are friendship and family so vital? Because the fear we experience is not simply of physical death and dying. There are deaths in abandonment, deaths in friendlessness, deaths in living without love, without passion, without purpose. Death and dying wear many disguises; life and recovery must call upon many allies. There is a profound correlation between illness and isolation, and between health and community.

In a Jewish tale the angels band together to conspire against God's intent to form Adam and Eve in His own image. They are jealous that ordinary men and women should inherit such spiritual treasure. The angels plot to hide goodness and truth from the human being. One angel proposes to hide God's mystery in the highest mountains; another suggests concealing it beneath the deepest seas. But the shrewdest angel counsels, "Men will search for godliness in the remotest of places. Hide it within them. It is the last place they will search for the miracles of godliness."

I received gifts of books in the hospital and during my recuperation. But I have come to learn what Buber concluded when he grew older. When in his youth he was asked which he preferred, Buber thought he preferred books to people. Books are easy to handle, easy to open and to close, to remove or place back on the shelves. Books are manna from heaven, while humans are like hard, brown bread on whose crust he breaks his teeth. But as he grew older, Buber changed his mind.

"I knew nothing of books when I came forth from the womb of my mother, and I shall die without books; I shall die with another human hand in my own."

What I fear, now that the energy returns, and the scars fade, is that I will forget the dark caverns of fear and those bright illuminations of love. There is, of course, a natural comfort in the mind's capacity to forget the fearful past; but the consolation would be questionable if loss of memory led to loss of gratitude. I now understand better the biblical imperatives to remember; to remember not only the Sabbath and the triumphs of the past, but the violations and defeats of our history; to remember the bondage in Egypt and villainy of the Amalekites so as to rejoice in our freedom and our strength. "Out of my depths, I have called unto God" (Psalms 130:1).

References

The Holy Scriptures. (1985). Philadelphia: Jewish Publication Society.

Midrash. (10 vols.). (1961). H. Freedman and M. Simons (Eds.). London: Soncino Press.

Shulchan Aruch. (10 vols.). (1965). New York: M.P. Press.

The Talmud. (18 vols.). (1961). I. Epstein (Ed.). London: Soncino Press.

Talmud (Jerusalem). (5 vols.). (1960). New York: Otzar Hasefarim.

PART II

FOUNDATION OF MEDICAL ETHICS

CHAPTER 4

THREE CARDINAL PRINCIPLES

OF JEWISH MEDICAL ETHICS

Rabbi Levi Meier, Ph.D.

The interface between health, medicine and Judaism encompasses the exploration of ethical issues in the maintenance of one's health and in its restoration and eventually, grappling with the inevitable. Jewish values and law are applied to the continuous development of scientific and technological advances in medicine.

Jewish medical ethics include both soft (psychosocial) and hard (medical) issues of the physician-patient relationship and the decision-making process. The soft issues reflect the dignity of all persons *qua* human beings regardless of their socio-economic status or quality of life. The dignity of the individual is beautifully summarized in the physician's prayer attributed to Moses Maimonides (1135-1204).

...Inspire me with love for my art and for Thy creatures. Do not allow thirst for profit, ambition for renown and admiration to interfere with my profession, for these are the enemies of truth and of love for mankind and they can lead astray in the great task of attending to the welfare of Thy creatures. Preserve the strength of

my body and of my soul that they ever be ready to cheerfully help
and support rich and poor, good and bad, enemy as well as friend.
In the sufferer let me see only the human being... (*The Bulletin of the
Johns Hopkins Hospital*, 28 [1917], pp. 256-61)

The hard issues require an analysis and ultimately, a resolution
among contrasting religious and secular value systems. The area of the
inception of life encompasses eugenics and genetics, Tay-Sachs disease,
test-tube babies, surrogate mothers, sex changes, contraception, abortion and
ritual circumcision. The area of the termination of life includes truth-telling,
euthanasia, resuscitation, organ transplantation, the definition of death and
autopsies.

Major Principles

Three major principles in Jewish medical ethics underlie Jewish legal
and moral premises relating to issues in medical ethics. These Jewish
principles are: human life has infinite value; aging, illness and death are a
natural part of life; and improvement of the patient's quality of life is a
constant commitment. All three principles are based on Biblical statements.

A.   **Human Life has Infinite Value.** The Bible states (Genesis
1:27) that God created the human being in the image of God, thus
differentiating human life from all other living matter. This uniqueness of
humanity is the basis of the principle that human life has *infinite* value.
This principle is a major axiom of Jewish medical ethics. Since infinity is
indivisible, even an infinitesimal fraction of a person's life is also of infinite
value. Human life or the value of human life is not dependent on any
external criterion. The value of human life is an absolute value.

B.   **Aging, Illness and Death are a Natural Part of Life.**

1. **Aging.** The aging process, from birth to death, represents
a normal, non-pathological unfolding of human development. Examples of
some normal age changes include a diminution in reaction time and a
postmenopausal decrease in gonadal hormones in men and women.
Although these physiological and other psychological and sociological
factors do change with time, aging is not a disease. A ninety-year-old
woman has the same right to life as someone nine or nineteen. Indeed,

aging is the anticipated blessing and reward for living an ethical and pious life (Exodus 20:12). Respect for the aged is prominently stated (Leviticus 19:32), and Rabbinic sages are frequently referred to as "elders." The Talmud (*Kiddushin* 32b) understands the word "aged" or "elderly" to epitomize mature wisdom of life experience. The absolute value of human life is not predicated on one's age, pragmatic utility or even upon the potential for service to one's fellow human being.

2. **Illness.** The inevitability of illness is a basic assumption of life. The Bible (Deuteronomy 4:9,15) places double emphasis on the necessary safeguards that one should take in caring for oneself. Whenever illness occurs, Judaism mandates that the patient seek medical assistance. As important as is the proper observance of all the Jewish laws, such as fasting on Yom Kippur (Day of Atonement) or the observance of the Sabbath, nevertheless proper care of one's physical and mental health always has priority when a person's health is threatened. Avoidance of the harmful becomes a religious commandment, subsumed under the guiding principle of taking good care of oneself (Deuteronomy 4:15). The *Shulhan Arukh* (Code of Jewish Law, *Orah Hayyim* 329:3) summarizes this thesis by stating that all laws of the Torah (except the cardinal three of idolatry, murder and forbidden sexual relations) are suspended when the possibility arises that one's life is in danger. Even hesitation in evaluating whether the danger to life is significant or not is deemed inappropriate.

The Bible (Exodus 21:19; Leviticus 19:16,18;25:35; Deuteronomy 22:2) grants specific permission and indeed mandates the physician to heal. In this manner, physician and patient become "partners with God," in attempting to conquer illness. At the end of the creation story (Genesis 2:3), God ceased from all His work which He had "*created to do.*" The *Midrash* (homiletical Biblical commentary, Genesis *Rabbah* 2:3) asks what is meant by the phrase "*created to do.*" The *Midrash* replies that God created the world with much more left to do. The work of creation is in a continuous process. When one creates by conquering illness, such as curing infections, one becomes a partner with God. According to Jewish tradition, the human response to illness is to be responsible for oneself and for one's neighbor. Health care was placed first by Maimonides among the ten important communal services that had to be offered by a city to its residents (*Mishneh Torah, Sefer HaMadda* IV:23).

**3.	Death.** Although the reality of death destroys the physicality of an individual, the idea of death confers meaning on life. An awareness of death moves one away from trivial preoccupations and concerns, and provides life with depth and substance from an entirely different perspective. The concept of death is also considered to be "good." "And God saw all that He had made and behold it was very good" (Genesis 1:31). The *Midrash* comments that the phrase "very good" includes death (Genesis *Rabbah* 9:5). Indeed, the dying process begins with birth. Rabbi Eliezer states (Mishnah, *Avot* 2:10): "repent one day before your death," to which the Talmud comments (*Shabbat* 153a): "Rabbi Eliezer's disciples asked him, 'Does one know when one is going to die?' He said to them, 'No, then certainly one should repent today, because maybe one will die tomorrow, thus, one will always be in the process of repenting.'"

Even when one is healthy, one can and should be aware that life is finite. A healthy awareness of life's finiteness should constantly lead one to search for a meaningful existence. A terminal illness only accentuates the reality and imminence of death and urges a more acute focus on the duration of time left before one dies. If there were no death, there would be no illness or aging. Succinctly stated, without death there is no life.

The exact time of one's death is not known beforehand. This fact is part of the gift of life and gift of death. It is both the known and the unknown which together endow life with the potential for finding meaning. The known aspect is that death is the common denominator of all of humankind; the unknown is the exact time of death. These together allow death to constantly endow life with meaning.

The Bible states the reason why life is finite. The Bible states: "And God said: My spirit shall not be in man forever, since he is also composed of flesh; and his days shall be one hundred-and-twenty years" (Genesis 6:3). God specifically created human beings with diametrically opposed entities, spirit and flesh, which cannot coexist eternally. God created people who would ultimately die. Death would then be a natural outgrowth of the lack of compatibility of flesh and spirit. Death is the natural outcome of life.

**C.	Improvement of the Patient's Quality of Life is a Constant Commitment.** One of the goals of the practice of medicine is to constantly improve the patient's quality of life. Human beings are given the choice between life or death, blessing or curse, good or evil. The Bible commands that people opt to "choose life" (Deuteronomy 30:15-19). Jewish medical ethics are rooted in the doctrine of human responsibility. Within the limitations of heredity and environment, everyone is free to choose order over chaos, homeostasis over disequilibrium, and family over a life of solitude. In Hebrew the word for life (*hayyim*) is always in the plural, representing the ultimate goal of life, which is living in tranquility with others.

Despite the fact that all medical and mental health professionals strive for the improvement of the patient's life, quality of life is never a factor in determining whether a patient should live or die. The sanctity of life is inviolable. Subjective considerations, either by the patient, physician or family, cannot allow either homicide, suicide or fratricide (Genesis 9:5). The reality of pain, suffering and anguish requires compassion, support groups, pain medication and whatever else may ameliorate the patient's condition, but not the termination of the life. Naturally, this approach does not preclude the patient's choice to refuse further treatment if the risk-benefit ratio is not favorable and if such treatment may hasten the patient's death.

Implications

Every medical-ethical dilemma requires its own analysis and resolution. However, based on the previous three major principles of Jewish medical ethics, two examples, one from the beginning of life and one from the end of life, will be offered on how these principles are operationalized in real situations.

Abortion

An abortion, the killing of potential human life, is allowed and even mandated if the life or health of the mother is gravely threatened. However, for most other reasons, an abortion is prohibited. The stated rationale for this ruling (Mishnah, *Oholot* 7:6) is that the mother's actual life takes precedence over the *potential* human life of the fetus. This overriding concern for the welfare of the mother is prior to the birth of the fetus. From the moment of birth, the value of both the infant's and the mother's life is absolute.

Euthanasia

Since the human being is created in the image of God, its life is sacred. It may not be terminated because of considerations of the patient's suffering. Suicide and euthanasia are both prohibited under the category of homicide. A physician is committed to prolonging the life of a patient and trying to cure the patient. It makes no difference whether the life prolonged is of long or short duration. An exception is made (permitting passive euthanasia) only for the case of a patient who is defined by Jewish law as moribund, i.e., for whom the death process has actually begun. Euthanasia, even when it is motivated by compassion (designed to put an end to unbearable pain), is tantamount to murder (Genesis 9:5). Naturally, everything should be done to alleviate the patient's suffering (Leviticus 19:18) save sacrificing a life.

References

The Holy Scriptures. (1985). Philadelphia: Jewish Publication Society.

Maimonides, M. (12th century) (1962). *Mishneh Torah* (6 vols.). New York: M.P. Press.

The Midrash. (10 vols.). (1961). H. Freedman & M. Simon (Eds.) London: Soncino Press.

Shulhan Arukh. (10 vols.). (1965). New York: M.P. Press.

The Talmud. (18 vols.). (1961). I. Epstein (Ed.). London: Soncino Press.

CHAPTER 5

ON BEING A JEWISH PHYSICIAN

Robert E. Levine, M.D.

Introduction

For thousands of years, the physician has occupied a special place in Judaism. The list of prominent Jewish thinkers who were also physicians includes Asaph, Maimonides, Nahmanides and many others. Any listing of prominent physicians, down to our present time, includes a percentage of Jews far greater than would be expected on the basis of the general world population.

What is the nature of the relationship between Judaism and medicine, and what does it mean both in theoretical and practical terms today to a Jew who is also a physician? My answers should be construed as personal ones, based on the nearly three decades of experience I have had in medicine since I entered medical school.

The Study of Medicine as a Religious Experience

The typical premedical student takes at least two years of chemistry, a year of physics and a year of zoology as an undergraduate. Yet, it is not until medical school that the mysteries of the nature of life are unraveled in meticulous detail, and in that unraveling, the religious mind begins to understand the distinction between the finite and the Infinite. It is one thing to think about evolution in simplistic generalities. It is quite another to be confronted by the molecular biology of a single cell whose intricacies surpass our understanding. Yet, at the medical school level one gains enough of an understanding of that cell to realize that it must represent the perfection of a master plan, not of a series of random happenings.

What can be said of the elegance of molecular biology is compounded as one learns about each organ, and the relationship of those organs to each other to make up the human organism. Direct involvement with the process of birth and recovery from illness begins to give human understanding to the Divine term, "miracle."

We are told in Exodus 33:18-23 how Moses asked to see God and was allowed to see only His back. Many of the commentaries interpret this to mean that Moses saw some manifestation of God. I doubt if -- since the days of Moses and the later prophets -- any group of Jews has had a better opportunity for seeing the manifestations of the Divine more clearly or more intimately than those who are privileged to be physicians. Beginning with their studies of anatomy and molecular biology, and continuing with their ongoing interactions with patients, physicians bear daily witness to the manifestation of the Divine in this world.

How the Physician Views God and Humanity

As the body of knowledge of medicine grows, so must the awe with which the physician views the human body, and in turn, the Creator of that human. Further, the human is viewed as *tzelem Elohim,* created in the image of God.

As one can dismantle a violin into its smallest elements and find no music, so one can dissect the human organism and find no soul. Yet, the physician is keenly aware of the existence of the special characteristics which define an individual and which are the earthly determinants of the soul. That awareness is the product of the vicarious living of many lives, the experience of the physician who is involved with patients and their problems.

In summary, the physician has an ever-increasing awe for the Creator, and for what has been created, the body and the soul. This awe is the basis for defining the special relationships between the physician, God and humanity that in turn define how a Jewish physician practices medicine.

How the Patient Views the Jewish Physician

When I was on duty as an intern in the Mount Sinai Hospital of New York emergency room, I attended an elderly Jewish patient in severe congestive heart failure. When she first came in, her breathing was so labored that she was unable to speak. As her treatment progressed, and she regained her ability to speak, her first sentence to me was, "I would like you to meet my granddaughter."

On the surface, the episode described could be interpreted as nothing more than a grandmother's quest for a good marriageable prospect for her granddaughter. Going somewhat deeper, however, the encounter illustrates the special esteem in which the physician is held. An essential element of that esteem derives from the patient's view of the physician as one who is dedicated to the performance of *mitzvot*.

Mitzvot are loosely thought of as "good deeds," but it is important to think of them in a more exact definition as "those acts which God wants done." In performing *mitzvot*, we are also imitating God. By practicing medicine, the physician is carrying out a number of *mitzvot* simultaneously: restoring lost health, analogous to the *mitzvah* of restoring a lost object to its owner (Deuteronomy 22:2) and not standing idly by while a fellow human is in trouble (Leviticus 19:16).

How Jewish Physicians Must View Themselves

The Jewish physician understands that his or her role is unique -- standing in the midst of the Divine plan of life, death and suffering, and having been given special permission by God to actively participate in that drama.

The text in Exodus 21:19 states that one who caused injury to another should cause the injured "to be thoroughly healed." Our tradition tells us that this specific phraseology is to be interpreted as permission for the physician to heal.

The physician, then, has the right to heal, and is performing *mitzvot* in so doing, even though we are told in Exodus 15:26 that healing comes from God. The physician must therefore feel himself or herself to be God's agent and to recognize that the physician's role is both markedly important and markedly limited. Further, as an agent, the physician must follow rules for job performance set by the Creator. These are the rules that are set out in *halakha,* the cumulative body of Jewish law.

Rashi (R. Solomon ben Isaac), the great commentator on the Torah, elaborates on Deuteronomy 22:8. The verse states: "When thou buildest a new house, then thou shall make a parapet for thy roof, that thou bring not blood upon thy house, if any man fall from thence." Quoting the *Siphre,* Rashi notes that good things are brought about through the agency of a righteous person, and bad things are brought about through the agency of one who is not righteous. The implication of this idea is that the better the moral character of the physician, the more likely he or she is to succeed as an agent for good, i.e., successful healing.

How *Halakha* Requires the Physician to Act

It is stated in Leviticus 18:5 that the Torah was given so that "you may live by it." We learn from that text that one is to live by the Torah, not die by it. The preservation of life, therefore, takes priority over all other considerations (except for the three cardinal sins of idolatry, forbidden sexual relationships and murder).

Sabbath restrictions and other religious laws must be set aside to save a life: the patient comes first. So many of the problems in the contemporary practice of medicine derive from failure to adhere to this basic principle. When considerations based on expedience, politics or economics come to the fore, the patient is no longer first, and unfortunately may even be last. It is the responsibility of the Jewish physician to keep the patient's interests first.

Although the physician must function within the *halakhic* framework, he or she bears the ultimate responsibility of deciding what is correct for the patient. In 1964, I was part of a small group of medical students who were meeting with the great *halakhic* authority of blessed memory, Rabbi Moshe Feinstein, to go over a number of practical medical *halakhic* problems. We were discussing the *halakhic* definition of fever which would categorize a critical illness for which other religious considerations could be suspended. At one point in the discussion he turned to us and said, "You are the doctors. If you think he is seriously ill, do what you need to do."

The concept that humans were created in the image of God teaches us that we must deal with our fellows with respect and dignity. This principle has special import in the practice of medicine because it is so easy for the patient to lose respect and dignity upon entering a hospital, to be thought of by a bed number or a diagnosis. He is no longer Mr. Smith. He is "the gallbladder in 603." The Jewish physician must never lose sight of the patient's individuality and unique needs.

Further, the concept that we are dealing with a human being who was created in the Divine image has another corollary. We may never say that there is nothing more to do for a patient, because there is always something more to do. Even if the patient's illness cannot be cured, or death prevented, there is still more to do. The Jewish physician is obligated to do all that is possible to ease that patient's pain, to allow him or her to retain dignity even in dying, and to help the family in any way that may be needed to deal with their crisis.

Lengthy volumes have been written on the specifics of how a Jewish physician must act in various situations, and we clearly cannot deal with all those *halakhic* cases in this chapter. Nevertheless, the foregoing has given us a broad outline of how to act:

- place the interests of the patient first
- assume the responsibility for caring for the patient and do whatever is necessary to help the patient
- treat the patient with respect and dignity
- never say there is no more that can be done.

Conclusion

We began by trying to understand the relationship between Judaism and medicine. In conclusion, we must realize that because of the interdependent relationship between the two, the better we strive to accomplish the dictates of one, the more we succeed in performing the other. For example, the more expert one is in one's medical practice, the more faithfully one has carried out the *mitzvah* of healing. Conversely, the more one appreciates the patient as created in the Divine image, and treats the patient accordingly, the better will be the quality of the medicine one practices.

Jewish physicians must continue throughout their lifetimes to upgrade their knowledge of the *halakhic* values which provide the framework for their medical skills, just as they continually upgrade those skills. Only in this way can they best serve their fellow humans, and in so doing, properly serve God.

CHAPTER 6

A CONCEPT OF ETHICS

Milton Heifetz, M.D.

Some of the important questions raised by students of ethics include: is there a single principle from which secondary principles may be derived and upon which decisions can rest, or are there multiple concepts of equal value which may be selectively used and applied to different situations and different circumstances? Is the basic frame of reference to be religious or secular? But the most important question that arises in any attempt to establish a moral framework is why one framework, principle or set of principles should be more readily accepted than any other.

In the Talmud, the writing of ancient Jewish sages, it is said that a man approached Shamai, a great teacher, and tauntingly asked him to explain the teachings of the whole Bible while the man stood on one leg. Shamai became incensed and rose to strike the stranger, who then ran to Hillel, the leader of the other main Rabbinical school and possibly the greatest sage of all. When asked the same question, Hillel stated,

> Do not to others that which you would not have others do to you. That is the whole Bible. The rest is commentary. Now go learn it.
> (Talmud, *Shabbat* 31a)

Hillel was not alone in expressing this thought as the essence of Hebraic philosophy. The same concept was widespread throughout the world. It is similarly stated in Hinduism as,

Do not unto others which would cause you pain if done to you. (Mahabarata 5, 1517)

In Buddhism, it is expressed as,

Hurt not others in ways that you yourself would find hurtful (Udana-Varga 5, 18)

In Confucianism, it is expressed as,

Do not unto others that which you would not have them do unto you. (Waley, 1983)

And in Zoroastrianism it is expressed as,

That nature alone is good which refrains from doing unto another whatsoever is not good for itself. (Dadistan-I-Dinik 94:5)

It was an integral part of Christianity during the early centuries (Hastings, 1914).

It was also expressed in ancient times outside of a religious context. Philo, a Roman emperor Alexander Severus, and the Greek writer Isocrates all used the same negatively stated principle. Henry More used it (Mead, 1965) and Hobbes reiterated it as a principle which anyone could understand (Hobbes, 1958).

This single concept appears to be the essence of the ethical philosophy of many religious and secular societies across the world.

It is probably the most universally accepted summary of the principles of human conduct.

What is the meaning of this axiom and what are its ramifications? Why is it considered so fundamental?

Let us analyze this *negatively* stated directive by asking: *What would we not have others do to us?*

Do not impose upon me. (Anything done to an individual which the individual does not desire or accept is an imposition.) This includes:

A. Do not physically hurt me or mine without my knowledge and consent.
B. Do not place burdens upon me or mine without my knowledge and consent.
C. Do not take anything from me or mine, whether tangible or intangible, without my knowledge and consent.
D. Do not invade my body, my home and my thoughts without my knowledge and consent.
E. Do not restrain, inhibit or prevent me from doing as I wish without my knowledge and consent.

This concept suggests that we would wish to be absolutely free to do anything we wish to do and still be free of harm. But since the principle must apply to all people, it is apparent that these two elements, freedom from harm and absolute freedom, are incompatible as a social doctrine. The resultant compromise and therefore the essence of Hillel's doctrine demands that *individual freedom is inviolate only as long as others are not harmed in the exercise of that freedom.* This concept of individual freedom, although qualified, is the essence of our sense of liberty.

There appears to be exquisite wisdom in this negatively stated concept. Love and benevolence are not ordered. Affection is not demanded. We cannot demand or legislate love, kindness, courtesy or respect, only civility and fairness. The directive was considered so fundamental because through this single concept, societies could live in harmony. The directive is reasonable, usable and livable.

But Hillel's final words, "now go learn it," suggest more than the cold, dispassionate axiom that one is free to act as long as one does not produce harm. The injunction to "learn it" exposes two additional concepts which are crucial and which permeate all secular and religious philosophy - the need to cooperate for the common good and beneficence.

The derivation of the "common good" factor from the negative Golden Rule is found in Hillel's admonition to "now go learn it." To learn it is to become aware that there is a hint of detachment, of separation from others in the concept "do not impose upon me." Separation can lead to destructive isolation. This implication had to be nullified, or at least softened by extending the concept of "do not impose upon me" to include "do not isolate me or mine," for surely harm will befall me or mine.

In essence, although common good is markedly altered by cultural influences and values which stress kindness and mutual concern, it appears to be, at the most fundamental level, tied to the desire to be free from harm. To implement these safety measures, rules and regulations arise which speak to the mutual obligations of the individual and the group; the ways in which each person must act for the group's benefit; and the group's obligations to the individual.

Beneficence, or altruistic behavior, may be defined as an action taken toward another person which is for the good of that person, regardless of whether that person is mature, competent, incompetent, conscious or unconscious. Its motivation is always honorable - to do good. It is the arm of benevolence. The key to whether an act or an attitude is benevolent is the *primary* intent to help even though the helper may also benefit from the act as a consequence.

The concept that you should love your neighbor as yourself (the "Golden Rule") appears once in the Old Testament (Leviticus 19:18) and was emphasized seven times in the New Testament. Although it is simply not reasonable to expect each person to love a neighbor or to give the neighbor whatever he would like his neighbor to give him, this principle intensified and extended the concept "do not harm" to an injunction to feel and show a sense of concern and kindness to others. Within the context of its formation, it stressed the need to avoid doing harm and to act with tenderness and compassion; to feel that sense of mutual concern which is the hallmark of a truly civilized society, a concern which has permeated all human thinking in spite of the evidence of hate, bigotry, intolerance, devastation and war that has marked our path.

The Golden Rule has a pervasive effect upon the attitude and actions of humanity. Without it, without our awareness of it and our attempt to at least partially live according to it, our lives would be colder, more detached and less humanized.

Changing circumstances or changing situations do not require new ethical values in order to be dealt with properly. Changing circumstances only demand a better understanding of basic principles and the ability to properly extrapolate those principles in changing times. The acceptance of multiple ethical values could too easily cause a gradual erosion of individual rights under the pretext of meeting communal needs, benevolence or so-called progress. At the same time we must not consider the basic framework as rigid rules, but as factors which need to be balanced. This approach is much less rigid than Kant's relatively firm demand that moral axioms be strictly followed. To negate the possibility of the need of a good lie would be absurd. To produce the harm that could ensue by telling the truth to a Gestapo agent would be a gross act of immorality.

One can find fault with any ethical framework. Any moral principle may be misused. I have a strong fear of misuse of social regulations. What is for the common good is subject to such a divergence of opinion that it may assume extremely dangerous, if not deadly aspects. Stalin's deadly program for the Soviet Union was conceived as best for the common good of all the Russians; Mao's Red revolution was also conceived as being warranted for the common good of China. These are but two examples of societal behavior patterns predicated upon a hierarchy which diminished individual freedoms to place the common good on the highest pedestal.

The essence of the United States Constitution lies in the understanding that the individual does not exist for the good of the state but the state for the individual. Its thrust is to insure a maximum of individual freedom. Fundamental to this thrust is the right of free choice in the absence of harm. This fundamental principle is congruent with, and derived from, the theological and secular concept, "Do not do to others that which you would not have done to you..." and most importantly it is consistent with patterns of mammalian behavior and human nature. The resultant factors form a framework of moral principles applicable to all situations involving ethics. The power behind this framework lies in its biological validity, or as Hobbes expresses it:

The laws of nature... need not any publishing nor proclamation, as being contained in this one sentence approved by all the world: Do not that to another which you think unreasonable to be done by another to yourself. (Hobbes, 1958)

There is a built-in risk within the hierarchy of this equation. An overemphasis placed upon personal freedom can lead to social inhumanity while undue importance given to the common good factor can lead to social tyranny. There is a balance which cannot be stipulated.

References

Hastings, J. (Ed.). (1914). *Encyclopedia of religion and ethics*. New York: Scribner's.

Hobbes, T. (1958). *Leviathan*. New York: Bobbs-Merrill.

The Holy Scriptures. (1985). Philadelphia: Jewish Publication Society.

Mead, F. (Ed.). (1965). *The Encyclopedia of religious quotations*. Westwood, N.J.: Revel.

The Talmud. (18 vols.). (1961). I. Epstein (Ed.). London: Soncino Press.

Waley, A. (Trans.). (1983). *The Analects of Confucius*. New York: Vintage Books.

CHAPTER 7

HUMAN DIGNITY AS REFLECTED IN THE

PHYSICIAN-PATIENT RELATIONSHIP:

A PHILOSOPHICAL JEWISH PERSPECTIVE

Rabbi David Hartman, Ph.D.

Recently, there was a public exchange of opinion between two physicians about organ transplants and the problem of the security of donors. The fact that an important hospital in New York was doing this very delicate surgery for people who were not citizens of the United States sparked the question: to whom do we owe responsibility? One of these physicians claimed that the essence of the medical profession is to deal with need, irrespective of communal identity, whereas the other argued, in a manner reminiscent of the Rabbinic saying that the poor of your own city come first (Deuteronomy 15:7, *Sifre* 116), that you should look after the needs of your own citizens. The dispute was related to a fundamental problem of ethics: to what degree does responsibility toward others grow from solidarity within a community, from some sort of social contract, from some sense of mutual claims that we can make upon each other, and to what degree does it grow from the essential dignity of every individual human being?

Another hotly discussed issue, certainly in Israel, is currently: where do we invest in medical research? Do we build more beds for the aged or do we develop our pediatrics department? Do we develop sophisticated equipment to deal with premature births, or do we find ways of alleviating the shame and disgrace that come with aging and the sense of isolation and loneliness that can envelop people in their final years?

I have mentioned these two examples in order to indicate that moral issues in medicine generally do not surface as simplistic conflicts between right and wrong, but as conflicts between one good and another.

Accordingly, the ethical dilemmas of the physician, as I once wrote in the *Journal of Medicine and Philosophy* (1979, volume 4, number 1), are not to be understood in terms of the quest for truth in a purely scientific sense in which one strives for certainty and for a knock-out argument that leads to a unique and necessary conclusion. The model of rational deliberation in medical ethics is more in the tradition of what Aristotle called *phronesis*, the tradition of practical reasoning. That is, one makes practical decisions using a form of deliberation which is such that one always remains aware that alternative decisions may also be reasonable. One can never have assurance that what one chose was necessary and the only rational position to maintain.

Thus, do you take care of your own community or do you take account of a universal framework? Do you respond to the aged or to the young? Do you view patients in terms of what you think their potential may be for the future of their social usefulness, or do you see each person in terms of intrinsic worth? Do you measure the value of life in terms of length or do you say, as Rabbi Jacob did, that "one hour of repentance and good deeds in this world is better than the whole world to come" (Mishnah, *Avot* 4:17)? How are you to quantify the quality of life, even if you want to use Bentham's principle of measuring happiness in terms of maximizing pleasure? How are you going to say that this person who has ten years is more significant than that person who has a day?

The Talmud repeatedly discusses the disputes between the school of Hillel and the school of Shammai (*Tannaim* during the first century). On page after page, these two academies point to different sensibilities, different approaches to the law. Finally, the Rabbis wanted to know who was right and they decided to go to the ultimate authority, the Sovereign of the Universe. After all, they were disputing about His Torah. He would know who interpreted it correctly. The heavenly voice answered: "These *and* these are the words of the living God" (Talmud, *Erubin* 13b). Both were in some way reflecting God's Torah.

This exemplifies an issue with which many scholars have dealt. Are there areas of thought where one cannot apply the law of contradiction, where there is no exclusive choice between A and not-A? We see that also in the Talmud, the theory of legal reasoning does not work with A and not-A.

Accordingly, even when the opinions of particular Rabbis were rejected, they were carefully preserved in the Mishnah, because the rejected opinion was not false, for when you decide according to the majority, it does not mean that the majority has discovered the truth, but that you are applying a procedural principle rather than a truth principle. The minority opinion is always recorded, because at some time in other circumstances this minority opinion may again surface and its approach may become the correct procedure for understanding Torah.

In other words, when you are dealing with life issues and trying to build meaning into human reality, when you are seeking not the true but the good - and unlike Plato, I distinguish between the two concepts - you are going to have to learn to live with profound anxiety. Consequently, those who deal with medical ethics have to take off their scientific epistemological caps and recognize that they have to be satisfied with Aristotle's *phronesis* and give up *theoria* - the concern with or search for certainty.

Two things make moral issues in medicine similar to *halakhic* (Jewish law) issues. One is that you are working within a context of scarcity. There are not sufficient resources for both the aged and the newborn in the lab. Second, doctors are faced with an urgency that a philosopher does not have. You are forced to make a decision; you cannot postpone judgment. The philosopher can take more time to deliberate, whereas the doctor has to decide within hours or minutes. How do I treat a cancer patient? Do I treat the illness or do I treat the total person? Do I administer drugs which may mar the person's sense of self-esteem and beauty or do I concentrate on alleviating pain? You have to make that decision in a context in which two values claim you.

It is situations of that kind which were debated so often in the Talmud. For instance (*Baba Mezia* 33a), who comes first - your father or your teacher? Whose lost object do you look for first? Whom do you help first when both are carrying heavy burdens? Whom do you ransom first? It was your father who brought you into this world, yet your teacher brings you into the world to come. Or, does that apply at most to one outstanding teacher, so that any other teachers certainly come after your father?

They ask this type of question because Talmudic ethics grows in a context of conflicts between one good and another. The Rabbis lived in a world of scarcity, a world where their decisions could always give rise to self-doubt and the possibility of being mistaken. If to be innocent is to be absolutely pure, then in such a world one is condemned to be guilty. But the search for that type of purity and certainty is illusory. It is an illusion to imagine that if we only knew all the facts and had enough time to weigh them, we would be able to come to a decision which would in some way be inevitable and necessary. However many facts and however much time one has, we cannot eliminate uncertainty. Therefore, I claim that the Talmud has much to offer medical ethics because it grapples with conflicts of your needs versus your parents' needs, your parents' needs versus your teachers' needs, your needs versus your wife's needs. How it seeks to balance one against the other may provide an interesting paradigm for contemporary medicine.

As we have grown in our capacity to enhance and enrich life, we have increasingly found that the very power which makes for enhancement also confronts us with grueling decisions concerning the proposed beneficiaries of our medical knowledge. Among some fine works relevant to these issues, I recommend a book by Michael Walzer called *Spheres of Justice* (Basic Books, 1983). In it, he continues the debate between Robert Nozick, who takes a libertarian position, and Bernard Williams, who takes a "need" position, in the dialectic of ideas about the nature of medicine: the guild idea, the market idea and the need idea. Against that backdrop, I shall try to clarify first what model I find within the Jewish philosophic tradition for the reality of medicine in a hospital setting, and then how I see the doctor-patient relationship within that conceptual model.

In *halakhic* (Jewish law) anthropology, be it from a Biblical, Rabbinic or Maimonidean perspective, there seems to be a polar tension in Judaism's understanding of the human condition. It is the polarity between *din*, justice, and *rahamim*, mercy. In the *Kabbalah* and in the *Midrash*, they are related to two Biblical names of the Divinity: respectively to *Elohim*, "God," and *Adonai*, "the Lord" - the Tetragrammaton. Regarding the first verse of the Bible, "In the beginning *Elohim* created the heaven and the earth," the Rabbis commented (Genesis *Rabbah* 12) that in the beginning, God thought to create the world on the principle of *din* alone. But when it comes to the creation of the first man (Genesis 2:7), the Biblical text reads "And *Adonai Elohim* created..." - both names of God are used. The *Midrash* therefore says: God saw that the world cannot live only by *din* and so He introduced *rahamim* as well.

To make the issue clearer, the word "justice" does not exhaust the Hebrew notion of *din*. The latter could also signify mutuality, demand, achievement, responsibility, initiative, the activist principle. Similarly, the Hebrew notion of *rahamim* does not mean merely mercy. It signifies the divine overflowing also associated with the term *hesed*, which is itself inadequately translated as "grace" or "lovingkindness." It is the principle whereby a human being is accepted unconditionally, whereby God responds to a person because he or she is. There is a confirmation of one's being and not merely a response to one's becoming; the person is seen not in terms of social role or activist stance or achievement orientation, but simply as being. One is loved, accepted and responded to because one is a human being.

Now these two poles, the rabbis recognized, constitute the rhythms through which we live out our existence. In terms of Greek thought, it is the polarity between the activist and the receptive principles, the active-passive contrast. Here passivity is not simply inactivity but a fundamental need in human consciousness. It is joy you feel in being, the joy you feel over your child because it is. Someone who has not intuited personal existence as worthwhile and did not experience the childhood joy of coddling, the joy of sensing that in someone else's eyes one's existence is intrinsically worthwhile, has missed a fundamental feature of what it means to become fully human. Human beings, who are created in the image of God, have intrinsic worth.

The essential worth of personhood is thus one feature of that polar experience. The other polar experience is the human being within an achievement-oriented framework, a person called upon to become. People are then thought of in terms of their potentials, their aspirations, their life-dreams. What have they made of their lives? Here human dignity is measured not by becoming; dignity is a social category, a creative challenge. You *become* dignified, you are not *born* dignified. You lack dignity unless you are able to assume responsibility for your own life, unless you are able to energize your own will, unless you are able to face the world with some sort of defiant posture, looking upon the world as a challenge. What can I do? How can I shape the world?

This shaping instinct, this call to become responsible, not just being but becoming, is the *din* principle. Both *din* and *rahamim* make up the human condition. Judaism did not decide for one principle alone. It therefore could not accept Paul's critique of the Mosaic law. Paul saw that God had made in the law at Sinai an unfulfillable demand, the source of a permanent uneasiness: can one ever truly fulfill one's responsibility? Guilt was therefore an accompanying feature of a law which made such enormous demands. Paul looked for liberation from those demands whereby he could intuit his existence to be worthwhile because of God's love.

We want to be certain of that love; we cannot bear to imagine that it is conditional. But God's demands in the law were seen as suggesting that His love was conditional. If you are using Erich Fromm's model, God is then the father who asks: "What have you become?" Or, it is like my mother's reaction when I wanted to feel important in some way and asked her about my *yihus* - my pedigree. She would answer: "It won't help you at all who your grandfather was." You have to create your own *yihus* - what you make of yourself.

The philosopher Martin Buber loved to tell a Hassidic story about someone called Zushia. When Zushia came to heaven, he was not asked why he had not been like the great Maimonides, why he had not been like some great saint. He was asked instead why during his life he had not been Zushia. Following Buber, people saw a deep humanism in this story. Surely it is wonderful that God is not going to ask me why I was not like Moses or Maimonides, because to read Maimonides is indeed to live with permanent guilt. When you see what he achieved, you must feel a tremendous sense of inadequacy. It is a kind of masochism to choose him as the philosopher to emulate. That is how I experience atonement in this unredeemed world.

In another sense, however, to ask me why I was not like Maimonides is not a difficult question. It is not paralyzing, since at least I know what *would* be expected of me. But to ask me why I was not David Hartman is actually the most terrifying question, for who has ever known what he could be?

I remember that once as a teenager I was given a poor rating in an intelligence test and my reaction was to feel that at least people might stop asking me: "Why don't you become somebody?" Yet there is something important behind that question, namely, that dignity is something you create. The activist pole, the call of aspirations, is essential, and not only the pole of compassion and acceptance. The love pole is only one aspect of the human condition; the achievement pole is also a vital feature of self-identity.

Now, where should medicine be placed in this bipolar framework? For in reality, there is social stratification and economic disparity. Recently we heard of the child who died because the hospital demanded $100,000 for heart surgery. Have we developed sophisticated frameworks to be able to cater only to the rich? When we discover how to prolong life, does that become a claim that all can make? Must we purchase medicine or does our need make us eligible for it? Must I buy medicine through my own social and economic achievements or inherited fortune, or must medical practitioners respond to me because I am in need, irrespective of my social and economic status?

In an emergency ward at the Hadassah Hospital in Jerusalem, an army captain, a student and an Arab worker are brought in. Whom do you treat first? Is treatment based upon a social perception of human worth, of who will contribute more to the society?

There are fields where we do give greater merit and honor and esteem to achievement, however needy the individual concerned may be. We do not award degrees at universities because "beloved is the human being created in the image of God" (Mishnah, *Avot* 3:14). Suppose I come forward and say: "I want a Ph.D. because my essential dignity depends upon it - because her parents won't let me marry her without it. Without this, they don't even want to look at me." They answer: "Fine, but in the university merit counts." Even those who want open enrollment at universities balk at giving degrees on demand.

My thesis - and Michael Walzer (1983) fundamentally saw that as well - is that there is no single principle of justice that can work in all frameworks of life. The tension between *din* and *rahamim* means that reality is never going to be monolithic. The quest for social integration is not going to be a harmonious whole, with one principle guiding all forms of behavior. Political communities are inevitably communities in conflict, where no uniform line can be drawn between the proper domains of the merit principle and the need principle. There is no Platonic form that could resolve that issue.

In large measure, we have to grope in the dark. Ours is an unredeemed world, meaning that we live inescapably in value conflict. We seek harmony as a desideratum but rarely achieve it. Therefore, what we ultimately do in human reality is that we build balances, we juggle between varying frameworks. When should a parent just hug the child and when should that parent say: "Get up on your feet and make a *mensh* (good person) of yourself?" When is it a time to speak and when a time to be silent? When is it a time to dance and when a time to weep? These questions in Ecclesiastes point not to a Stoic necessity, but to a polar movement between contrary possibilities. When does the doctor just stop and wait or accept defeat, and when does he or she go on trying again and again? How far does the will to change and create and explore dominate? At what point does it give way to silent resignation before a world that you cannot control?

Within that polar framework, I suggest that we expect the hospital to be a balance to social inequalities. Here, "beloved is the human being created in the image of God" is recognized as a normative principle. It feels counterintuitive that a person got better medical care because he or she was wealthy, that a person who came into the emergency ward was measured by his or her social productivity rather than essential being.

A hospital operates in the elemental domains of reality, where the *rahamim* principle should claim more weight than the activist *din*. Here the dominant principle is essence rather than social role. Whereas in many other domains of the totality of society, the merit principle of *din* holds its sway, here it is balanced by the *rahamim* principle. Medicine brings *rahamim* into social political reality. In coming inside the walls of a hospital, one intuitively needs to feel confirmed as a human being. One does not want at that moment to be reminded that one is poor or rich, black or white, Catholic or Protestant, Jew or Arab.

The Mishnah notes that "he who saves one life is as if he saved a whole world" (*Sanhedrin* 4:5), meaning that there are moments in human experience in which you validate the sacredness of human life outside of personal or collective historical memory. Those are moments in which my particularity does not define my attitudes to another human being. Although I love my brother, my mother and my people more than others, and although I am engaged much more with their needs, my moral experience must also have moments in which those aspects of my identity do not qualify my behavior, in which my solidarity with humanity becomes my *modus vivendi* - the ultimate claim upon myself.

A Kantian would ask whether I can universalize any particular moral decision that I make. There, I think Kant went too far. The criterion of universality is not the normative principle for all aspects of reality. There is also a place for what I would call responding to intimacy, family and community. Nonetheless, there are moments in which the intuitive confirmation of my solidarity with all of humanity plays the dominant role in my experience. Accordingly, the hospital situation, when it deals with this elemental value of human life, should reflect the *rahamim* principle rather than the *din* principle, despite all the familiar problematics that ensue. Insistence on *rahamim*, I also know, will not be a perfect solution and will not always be realizable. But I believe that it should be the ideal that the hospital contributes as one component of the moral, social and political framework of life. It is the balancing principle in a world in which achievement and merit dominate human identity.

I do not want to be understood, however, as suggesting that the dominant principle in *all* medical situations must be *rahamim* - mercy. So far we have been concentrating on the hospital situation where the patient is often desperate and helpless - literally at the mercy of those who are treating him or her. Many times when we focus on these desperate situations, we forget the enormously complex moral issues that arise in "ordinary" medical care. Perhaps the most fundamental issue in medicine is how a patient and a doctor build up a human relationship with each other over years of intermittent contact. That relationship may be far more complex and far more important to reflect upon than those acute issues which are philosophically interesting, but are not the predominant experience of most medical practitioners.

In the "ordinary" situations of the doctor-patient relationship, there is also important scope for the operation of *din*. Above all, it is *din* - doing "justice" to the patient - that requires the doctor to resist the paternalistic impulse to say: "Rely on me, patient, I will take care of you." On account of *din*, the doctor invites the patient to become responsible, such that the dignity of the patient is not subordinated to unquestioning trust in the physician, but flourishes as the patient is enabled to discover resources within the self to find ways of navigating through the hazards of life. Especially, the current renewal of emphasis on preventive medicine reflects the *din* principle, whereby you invite the community to become responsible for its own health.

Din is also the attempt not to infantilize the patient. It happens too often in Israeli medicine that you come in and the professor looks at you and says: "You don't have to speak; I know what's bothering you." This attitude resembles that of some Jewish mothers who used to tell their children: "I look at your forehead and I can see that someone gave you an evil eye." And then they would tell those children everything they had to do to get rid of the evil eye that had been directed at them. What I have learned from great physicians is their ability to ask the patient to help the doctor discover what kind of treatment is needed, their understanding that only in listening can one speak and that the hearing precedes the diagnosis. They invite the patient's help because "it will not be easy for me to be sure what is wrong with you unless you share with me your symptoms, share with me that which has been part of your life."

When building up a relationship, therefore, the doctor must offer a framework in which there is trust, for who wants to expose weaknesses even to a doctor? Who wants to be naked and to talk about symptoms to a stranger? There can be such a feeling of depersonalization in exposing one's nakedness, in exposing the lost illusion of one's sense of adequacy.

To invite someone to become dependent upon you is a great moral invitation that has to grow out of your ability to elicit trust.

Therefore, much depends on what happens at the moment of meeting, the moment when a patient just comes in, the first glance you give, the way the nurse greets the patient, the accuracy with which you give and keep appointments. I remember going to see an orthopedic surgeon somewhere in Jerusalem and found people who had been waiting there eight hours. There was such an atmosphere of anger, and yet nobody offered an apology, because you were seeing the great man who was going to take complete care of you when at last your turn came. So you were expected to appreciate what was being done for you, irrespective of minor inconveniences like sitting around waiting for a whole day.

When the first contact generates so much anger, you cannot then say, "Tell me what is wrong with you" and expect the person to speak uninhibitedly. By coming so late, therefore, the doctor has practiced medicine inadequately. I do not mean that he has not been a *mensh* (good person). It is not just a question of lack of humanity, since the professor was possibly showing great humanity to someone else and simply had not organized his schedule properly. The point is that unless you start doctor-patient relationships in a climate of trust, you practice bad medicine. For you are less likely to reach a proper diagnosis - if you can ever reach a proper diagnosis - unless there is that existential relationship of trust, which begins with the way people are welcomed in the hospital, the way they are talked to, the way their time is saved or wasted, the way their own human reality is respected in a strange environment. It is there that good medicine begins.

On the one hand, then, the *din* principle serves to invite the trusting framework of dependency, an environment where a person is not afraid to be naked. On the other hand, the doctor also needs to recognize - again without paternalism - those moments in which the patient finds it all too much. "Please, doc, work it out. Don't give me all the fifteen different possibilities that you could imagine. I can't handle all the complexities. Will you take care of me and don't involve me too much in what you are doing, because I am worn out and I would appreciate it very much if you would just carry me through my illness or hug me to the end, without involving me in every process." There are moments when the patient can only seek to be passive and to be taken care of, moments in which the doctor stands alone and has to make all the decisions.

There is a tendency in patients toward psychological regression in illness. It should not always be seen in a bad sense. During illness, there may come the desire to recapture that primordial moment of coddling, that primordial moment when someone just hugs you because you are. There is that sense of being taken care of, that intuition that I am cared for, loved in my weakness. That may be a genuine need in any patient at certain moments. The great danger of illness is that a person chooses to remain ill because he or she cannot deal with the *din* principle. Since we love the *rahamim* principle, we sometimes fight and get angry at the physician who says, "You can go home!"

What does it mean when you say to a person: "You can go home"? You are telling someone to go back again into the *din* world, back into the world of merit and achievement. Therefore, you will find patients constantly coming back just because what they seek is to remain in the childlike atmosphere of *rahamim*, of grace, in which distinctions between people are not made and one's existence is intuited as worthwhile, independent of achievement.

Maimonides writes that a man "who cannot live without help but who, in his pride, declines to accept help is a shedder of blood, guilty of attempts on his own life" (*Mishneh Torah, Hilkhot Tzedakah* 10:19). But before that, he makes the opposite point: "He who, having no need of alms, obtains alms by deception, will fall into a dependency that is real before he dies of old age" (*ibid*). To choose dependency when one can be personally adequate is to destroy a fundamental vision of the Jewish tradition that dignity is a category of achievement and responsibility. It is a category of *mitzvah*, of divine commandment, of demand. Medicine, too, should in some way invite the person to that form of responsibility.

As these quotations from Maimonides indicate, both fear of dependency and fear of responsibility lead to a dwarfed life. So when the dialectic of doctor-patient relationship moves between the poles of *din* and *rahamim*, which gets greater weight in the Jewish tradition? Is it fifty-fifty? Maimonides implies that if you are in pain, push self-reliance as far as you can. Hold to the *din* principle. But when you cannot work it out, then call for *rahamim*. For ultimately, in Jewish ethics, God's presence is felt when the community feels dignified in assuming responsibility for the covenantal drama of Israel.

References

Hartman, D. (1979). Moral uncertainties in the practice of medicine: The Dynamics of interdependency from a *Halakhic* perspective. *The Journal of Medicine and Philosophy*, 4(1), 98-112.

The Holy Scriptures. (1985). Philadelphia: Jewish Publication Society.

The Midrash. (10 vols.) (1961). H. Freedman & M. Simon (Eds.) London: Soncino Press.

Sifre. In Malbim, M. (19th century). (1964). Commentary to the Pentateuch: Deuteronomy. New York: Grossman.

The Talmud. (18 vols.) (1961). I. Epstein (Ed.). London: Soncino Press.

Walzer, Michael. (1983). *Spheres of justice.* New York: Basic Books.

CHAPTER 8

THE PATIENT-PHYSICIAN RELATIONSHIP:

RESPONSIBILITIES AND LIMITATIONS

Fred Rosner, M.D.

Introduction

Jewish medical ethics is based on the concept of the infinite value of human life. As a result all efforts must be applied to heal the sick, to cure illness and to prolong life. Even the Sabbath and Yom Kippur must be desecrated to save a human life, and all biblical and rabbinic rules and regulations except the cardinal three must be suspended in the face of danger to life. These three exceptions are idolatry, murder and forbidden sexual relationships such as incest. Even a few moments of life are worthwhile. Judaism is a "right to life" religion. The obligation to save lives is both an individual and a communal obligation. A physician is divinely licensed and biblically mandated to use medical skills to heal the sick and thereby prolong and preserve life. A patient is morally bound and biblically mandated to seek healing from a physician.

How far does the physician's obligation to heal extend? Is the physician obligated to endanger his own life to treat patients with contagious and/or communicable diseases? How much risk to their own health and lives are physicians allowed or obligated to undertake in the care of their patients? How far does the patient's obligation to seek healing extend? Is a terminally ill patient obligated to accept all medical therapies to the very end? Is the patient obligated to follow the physician's advice? Is the patient mandated to allow resuscitative efforts for cardiopulmonary arrest?

The Physician's License and Obligation to Heal

The ethical and legal question of whether or not a person is allowed in Jewish law to become a physician and heal the sick is based on the biblical statement in which God asserts: *I am the Lord that heals you*[1] which literally translated from the Hebrew means I am the Lord, your physician. If God states that He is the Healer of the sick, how can we, as human physicians, play God, so to speak?

Various interpretations are offered to explain this scriptural verse. In his biblical commentary, Rashi explains *I am the Lord that heals you* to mean that God teaches the laws of the Torah in order to save man from disease. Rashi uses the analogy of a physician who tells his patient not to eat such and such a food lest it bring him into danger from disease. So too, continues Rashi, obedience to God's commandments is *health to your body and marrow to your bones*[2]. In a similar vein, the extratalmudic collection of biblical interpretation known as the *Mechilta* asserts that the words of Torah are life as well as health, as it is written: *they are life unto those that found them and health to all their flesh*[3]. Other commentators extend this thought by propounding that the Divine Law restores health and certainly prevents illness from occurring, thus serving as preventive medicine against all physical and social evil. The commentator known as *Malbim* interprets the phrase *I am the Lord that heals you* to include mental or spiritual illness and that God's statutes are for our benefit, not His.

The multitude of interpretations of the scriptural verse *I am the Lord that heals you* indicates that this phrase is not to be understood literally. There is no absolute prohibition inherent in this verse preventing a person from becoming a physician and healing the sick. In fact, specific permissibility, sanction and even mandate for the physician to practice medicine is given in the Torah, based on the rabbinic interpretation of the biblical phrase *and heal he shall heal*[4]. The Sages in the Talmud interpret the duplicate mention of healing in the phrase *heal he shall heal* to mean that authorization was granted by God to a physician to heal[5]. The Bible implies that it is as if there are two physicians; one is Almighty God, the true Healer of the sick, and the other is the human physician who serves as an instrument of God or an extension of God in the ministrations to the sick.

Many biblical commentators echo this talmudic teaching. By the insistence or emphasis expressed in the double wording, the Bible opposes the erroneous idea that having recourse to medicine shows lack of trust and faith in divine assistance. The Bible takes it for granted that medical therapy is used and actually requires it.

Moses Maimonides derives the biblical sanction for a physician to heal from the scriptural commandment *and thou shalt restore it to him*[6] which refers to the restoration of lost property. In his Mishnah commentary, Maimonides asserts:

> It is obligatory from the Torah for the physician to heal the sick and this is included in the explanation of the scriptural phrase *and thou shalt restore it to him*, meaning to heal his body[7].

Thus, Maimonides states that the law of the restoration of a lost object also includes the restoration of the health of one's fellow man. If a person has "lost his health" and the physician is able to restore it, he is obligated to do so. Maimonides's reasoning is probably based upon a key passage in the Talmud which states: "whence do we know that one must save his neighbor from the loss of himself? From the verse *and thou shalt restore it to him*." Thus even if someone is attempting suicide or refuses treatment for illness, one is obligated to intervene to save the person's life and health.

The second scriptural mandate for a physician to heal is based on the phrase *do not stand idly by the blood of your neighbor*[8]. This passage refers to the duties of human beings to one another. One example cited in the Talmud is the following:

> Whence do we know that if a man sees his neighbor drowning or mauled by beasts or attacked by robbers, he is bound to save him? From the verse *do not stand idly by the blood of your neighbor*[9].

Maimonides codifies this talmudic passage in his famous Code of Jewish Law known as *Mishneh Torah* as follows:

> Whoever is able to save another and does not save him transgresses the commandment *do not stand idly by the blood of your neighbor*. Similarly, if one sees another drowning in the sea, or being attacked by bandits, or being attacked by a wild animal and is able to rescue him...and does not rescue him...he transgresses the injunction *do not stand idly by the blood of your neighbor*[10].

Such a case of drowning is considered as loss of one's entire body and one is obligated to save it. Certainly one must cure disease which often afflicts only part of the body.

In summary, it is evident in Jewish tradition that divine license is given to a physician to heal, based on the interpretation of the biblical phrase *heal he shall heal*. Many Jewish scholars such as Maimonides claim that healing the sick is not only allowed but is obligatory. Joseph Karo's famous Code of Jewish Law known as *Shulchan Aruch* seems to combine both thoughts:

> The Torah gave permission to the physician to heal; moreover, it is a religious precept and is included in the category of saving life; and if he withholds his services, it is considered as shedding blood[11].

The Patient's Obligation to Seek Healing

It is clear from the aforementioned that a physician is divinely licensed and biblically obligated to heal the sick because of the Jewish concept of the supreme value of human life. Is a patient, however, authorized or perhaps mandated to seek healing from a physician? Is a patient who asks a physician to heal him denying Divine Providence? Is a person's illness an affliction by God that serves as punishment for wrongdoing? Does one forego atonement for one's sin by not accepting the suffering imposed by Divine Judgment and seeking medical care from a physician? Is there a distinction between heavenly afflictions and man-induced illness or injury?

The strongest evidence in Jewish sources that allows and even mandates a patient to seek healing from a physician is found in Maimonides's *Mishneh Torah* as follows:

A person should set his heart that his body be healthy and strong in order that his soul be upright to know the Lord. For it is impossible for man to understand and comprehend the wisdoms [of the world] if he is hungry and ailing or if one of his limbs is aching...[12]

He also recommends[13], as does the Talmud[14], that no wise person should reside in a city that does not have a physician. Maimonides's position is further expanded and codified as follows:

Since when the body is healthy and sound [one treads] in the ways of the Lord, it being impossible to understand or know anything of the knowledge of the Creator when one is sick, it is obligatory upon man to avoid things which are detrimental to the body and to acclimate himself to things which heal and fortify it[15].

There are numerous talmudic citations which indicate that patients when sick are allowed and even required to seek medical attention. One who is in pain should go to a physician[16]. If one is bitten by a snake, a physician is called even on the Sabbath because all restrictions are set aside for possible danger to human life[17]. If one's eye is afflicted, one may prepare and apply medication even on the Sabbath[18]. Rabbi Judah the Prince, compiler of the Mishnah, suffered from an eye ailment and consulted his physician, Mar Samuel, who cured the ailment by placing a vial of chemicals under the rabbi's pillow so that the powerful vapors would penetrate the eye[19]. In the case of bodily injury, if the offender tells the victim that he will bring a physician who will heal for no fee, the victim can object and say: "a physician who heals for nothing is worth nothing[20]."

From these and other talmudic passages, it is evident that an individual is not only allowed, but probably required to seek medical attention when he is ill. In Jewish tradition, the patient is obligated to care for his health and life. He is charged with preserving his health. He must eat and drink and sustain himself and must seek healing when he is ill in order to be able to serve the Lord in a state of good health.

The Physician's Obligation to Heal Patients with Contagious Diseases

Having established the physician's divine mandate to heal the sick, one can ask: how far does this mandate extend? Is a physician obligated to treat a patient with a contagious disease if there is a risk that the doctor may contract the illness from the patient? Is a physician obligated to endanger his own health or life to restore the health and/or save the life of the patient?

I have already mentioned that Jewish law requires that if one sees one's neighbor drowning or mauled by beasts or attacked by robbers, one is bound to save him. This rule is codified by Maimonides[21] and Karo[22]. Elsewhere, Karo rules[23] that if one observes a ship sinking with people on board, or a river flooding over its banks thereby endangering lives, or a pursued person whose life is in danger, one is obligated to desecrate the Sabbath to save them. The commentaries add that if there is danger involved to the rescuer, the latter is not obligated to endanger his life because his life takes precedence over that of his fellow man. If there is only a small risk (*sofek sakanah*) to the rescuer, he should carefully evaluate the small risk or the potential danger to himself and act accordingly.

What should a physician do if his patient is suffering from a contagious disease which the physician might contract? Is the physician allowed to refuse to treat the patient because of the risk or the fear by the physician of contracting the disease? What if the risk is very small (*sofek sakanah*)? What is the definition of small risk? If there is a greater than fifty-percent chance of the physician contracting the disease from his patient, Jewish law would certainly agree that such odds are unacceptable and the physician would not be obligated to care for that patient without taking precautionary measures to protect himself. If he wishes to do so in spite of the risk, his act is considered to be a pious act (*midat chasidut*) by some writers and folly (*chasid shoteh*) by others. But if the risk is very remote, the physician must care for that patient.

The question as to whether or not a person is obligated or allowed to subject himself to a risk in order to save another person's life is related to the well-known difference of opinion between the Babylonian and Jerusalem Talmuds. The latter[24] posits that a person is obligated to potentially endanger his life (*sofek sakanah* or small risk) to save the life of another from certain danger (*vadai sakanah* or great risk). On the other hand, the Babylonian Talmud[25] voices the opinion that a person is not obligated to endanger his life even if the risk is small, in order to save the life of another.

The prevailing opinion among the various rabbinic sources is the one cited by Rabbi David Ibn Zimra, known as Radvaz[26]. If there is great danger to the rescuer, he is not allowed to attempt to save his fellow man; if he nevertheless does so, he is called a pious fool. If the danger to the rescuer is small and the danger to his fellow man very great, the rescuer is allowed but not obligated to attempt the rescue, and if he does so his act is called an act of lovingkindness (*midat chasidut*). If there is no risk at all to the rescuer or if the risk is very small or remote, he is obligated to try to save his fellow man. If he refuses to do so, he is guilty of transgressing the commandment *thou shalt not stand idly by the blood of thy fellow man*[27]. This approach is also adopted by recent rabbinic decisors including Rabbi Moshe Feinstein[28] and Rabbi Eliezer Yehuda Waldenberg[29]. If the risk to physicians and other health personnel in caring for patients with contagious diseases such as tuberculosis or communicable diseases such as the acquired immunodeficiency syndrome (AIDS) is very small, a physician is obligated in Jewish law to care for such patients. The risk of contracting AIDS from a needle stick from AIDS virus infected blood is less than one-percent.

Let me dwell for a few moments on the physician's obligation to care for AIDS patients. Medical history and tradition are replete with examples of physicians whose devotion to their patients transcended any possible personal danger of contracting their patients' disease. Physicians caring for patients with plague, cholera, typhoid and polio occasionally became victims themselves.

Throughout the ages, physicians' obligations not only to their patients but to society, other health professionals and to themselves have not always been accepted as axiomatic. The profound reluctance of some physicians to care for patients with AIDS prompted Zuger and Miles[30] to review medical responses to other historic plagues. Many physicians, including Galen from Rome in the second century and Sydenham from London in the seventeenth century, fled from patients with contagious epidemic diseases. Yet, many of their colleagues, at considerable personal risk, remained behind to care for plague victims.

The Council on Ethical and Judicial Affairs of the American Medical Association (AMA) stresses the doctor's duty to AIDS patients[31] by stating that:

- A physician may not ethically refuse to treat a patient whose condition is within the physician's current realm of competence solely because the patient is seropositive.

- Physicians are dedicated to providing competent medical service with compassion and respect for human dignity.

- Physicians who are unable to provide the services required by AIDS patients should make referrals to those physicians or facilities equipped to provide such services.

The American College of Physicians and the Infectious Diseases Society of America believe that physicians, other health care professionals and hospitals are obligated to provide competent and humane care to all patients, including patients with AIDS and AIDS-related conditions, as well as HIV-infected patients with unrelated problems. The denial of appropriate care to patients for any reason is unethical[32].

The Association of American Medical Colleges adopted a statement concerning the professional responsibility in treating AIDS patients which, in part, stated that:

Medical students, residents, and faculty have a fundamental responsibility to provide care to all patients assigned to them, regardless of diagnosis. A failure to accept this responsibility violates a basic tenet of the medical profession--to place the patient's interest and welfare first[33].

Yet, in spite of the pronouncements of these and other august bodies, physicians are not saints, but healers. Neither law nor ethics expects sainthood or martyrdom of health care professionals, nor can the law force people to be courageous or virtuous[34]. The professional obligation of a physician based on the devotion to the moral ideal of healing the sick has some qualifications. Physicians are obviously not obligated to treat patients whose diseases are outside their area of competence. Other limiting factors include excessive risk, minimal or questionable benefits, competing obligations to other patients, and competing obligations to self and family[35].

The overwhelming consensus of opinion seems to be that men and women assume a unique responsibility when they enter a healing profession. "Having accepted the mantle of a doctor, we are no longer absolutely free to choose which patients we will and will not treat[36]." Medicine is different from business and most other careers and, therefore, imposes an obligation of effacement of self-interest on the physician. These differences of "the nature of illness, the nonproprietary character of medical knowledge, and the oath of fidelity to the patient's interests, generate strong moral obligations[37]."

The Physician's and Patient's Responsibilities in Terminal Illness

How does one treat or not treat a terminally ill patient who is close to death? Should the patient be fed and washed? Should the patient be given oxygen if needed? Should the patient be treated with antibiotics for pneumonia? Should the patient be given blood transfusions for hemorrhage? Should the patient be subjected to surgery for acute appendicitis or a perforated peptic ulcer? Should the patient be intubated and/or placed on a respirator for respiratory distress? Should the patient be resuscitated following cardiorespiratory arrest? Where does one draw the line?

One basic question seems to be the extent to which individuals own their own death. Do people have the right to select how and when they will die? Is such a decision by the patient akin to suicide? To what extent are individuals responsible for their own lives and health? Judeo-Christian teaching is that life is a gift of God to be held in trust. One is duty bound to care for one's life and health. Only God gives life and hence only God can take it away. This individual responsibility for the preservation of one's life and health is apart from the duty of one person (including a physician) toward another's life and health, and society's responsibility concerning the life and health of its citizens.

The doctor-patient relationship is no longer what it used to be because of a variety of factors. There are legal forces, such as the medical malpractice issue, that may interfere with the physician's best clinical and ethical judgment. There are psychological forces pushing the physician to "do something." There are professional forces that may force a physician to act to protect himself from peer review. Patients are better informed and becoming more vocal. Physicians' own religious and ethical values, their own experiences, their teaching by preceptors all play a role in deciding how they approach a dying patient. Ultimately, to whom are physicians responsible? To themselves? To the patient? To society? Or to God?

The infinite value of human life in Judaism means that one moment of life is of equal value to one minute or one hour or one day or one week or one month or one year or a decade or seventy years of life.[38] Even in the final phase of life, the Talmud clearly states that "one who closes the eyes of a dying person while the soul is departing is a murderer. This may be compared to a lamp that is going out. If a man places his finger upon it, it is immediately extinguished[39]." The small effort of closing the eyes may slightly hasten death.

Rabbi Eliezer Yehuda Waldenberg states that physicians and others are obligated to do everything possible to save the life of a dying patient, even if the patient will live for only a brief period, and even if the patient is suffering greatly[40]. Any action that results in hastening the death of a dying patient is forbidden and considered an act of murder. Even if the patient is beyond cure and is suffering greatly and requests that his death be hastened, one may not do so or advise the patient to do so[41]. A terminally ill patient may be given oral or parenteral narcotics or other powerful analgesics to relieve his pain and suffering, even at the risk of depressing his respiratory center and hastening his death, provided the medications are prescribed solely for pain relief and not to hasten death[42].

Waldenberg also states that it is not considered interference with the Divine Will to place a patient on a respirator or other life-support system. On the contrary, all attempts must be made to prolong and preserve the life of a patient who has a potentially curable disease or reversible conditions. Thus, one must attempt resuscitation on a drowning victim who has no spontaneous respiration or heartbeat because of the possibility of resuscitation and reversibility. One is not obligated or even permitted, however, to initiate artificial life support and/or other resuscitative efforts if it is obvious that the patient is terminally and incurably and irreversibly ill with no chance of recovery. One is also allowed to disconnect and discontinue life support instrumentation if one can establish that the patient is dead according to Jewish legal criteria[43], that is, if the patient has no independent brain function or spontaneous cardiorespiratory activity[44]. If it is not clear whether the respirator is keeping the patient alive or only ventilating a corpse, the respirator must be maintained. It may not be turned off to test whether the patient has spontaneous respiratory activity because that small act may be the one that causes the patient's death, similar to the flickering lamp which may be extinguished if someone touches it. Finally, Rabbi Waldenberg asserts that blood transfusions, oxygen, antibiotics, intravenous fluids, oral and parenteral nutrition, and pain-relief medications must be maintained for a terminally ill patient until the very end.

Rabbi Shlomo Zalman Auerbach also states that a terminally ill patient must be given food and oxygen even against his will[45]. However, one may withhold, at the patient's request, medications and treatments which might cause him great pain and discomfort. Auerbach also distinguishes between routine and nonroutine treatments for the terminally ill. For example, a dying cancer patient must be given food, oxygen, antibiotics, insulin, and the like, but does not have to be given painful and toxic chemotherapy which offers no chance of cure but at best temporary palliation. Such a patient may be given morphine for pain even if it depresses his respiration. An irreversibly ill terminal patient whose spontaneous heartbeat and breathing stop does not have to be resuscitated.

Rabbi Moshe Hershler opines that withholding food or medication from a terminally ill patient so that he dies is murder[46]. Withholding respiratory support is equivalent to withholding food, since it will shorten the patient's life. Every moment of life is precious, and all measures must be taken to preserve even a few moments of life. However, if the physicians feel that a comatose patient's situation is hopeless, they are not obligated to institute life-prolonging or resuscitative treatments.

Rabbi J. David Bleich affirms that although euthanasia in any form is forbidden, and the hastening of death, even by a matter of moments, is regarded as tantamount to murder, treatment may be withheld from the moribund patient (*goses*) in order to provide for an unimpeded death[47]. While the death of a *goses* may not be hastened, there is no obligation to perform any action which might lengthen the life of such a patient.

The most extensive discussion in the recent rabbinic literature of the treatment of the terminally ill is that of Rabbi Moshe Feinstein[48] who, in the seventh volume of his famous responsa *Iggrot Moshe*, states that for a patient with pain and suffering who cannot be cured and cannot live much longer, it is not obligatory for physicians to administer medications to briefly prolong his life of pain and suffering, but nature may be allowed to take its course. However, it is prohibited to give the patient any medication or do any act to hasten his death by even a moment. Pain relief medications, however, should always be administered as necessary.

A terminally ill patient with respiratory difficulties should be given oxygen even if he cannot be cured, because oxygen relieves discomfort, continues Feinstein. Rabbi Feinstein also points out that care must be exercised not to unnecessarily touch a dying patient, as discussed earlier in this essay. A person in whom death is imminent (*goses*) may not be touched or moved unnecessarily lest this act hasten the patient's death. Many Jewish as well as non-Jewish physicians are either not aware of or concerned about this prohibition, decries Feinstein. However, in Jewish law, hastening a person's death by even a moment is considered an act of murder. Touching the patient as part of his medical or supportive care is obviously not only permissible, but mandatory.

The use of dangerous medications for the terminally ill is discussed by Rabbi Feinstein as follows: Although the danger of a medication may be far less than the danger of an illness, physicians should carefully weigh whether this is true not only for relatively strong patients or for those with non-dangerous illnesses, but also for those who are gravely ill. Only if physicians know that the risk of the side effects of a medication are minimal in a gravely ill patient, or more than half such patients are cured, should they administer that medication and even then, only with the patient's consent. Such difficult decisions should be discussed and made by a group of physicians and not by a single physician.

The treatment of an intercurrent illness in a terminally ill patient is addressed by Rabbi Feinstein as follows: If a patient with a painful incurable illness (such as metastatic cancer) develops an intercurrent illness which is treatable and often completely reversible (such as pneumonia or urinary tract infection), it is obligatory to treat the intercurrent illness. However, if the underlying incurable disease is very painful and the patient refuses additional palliative therapy, it is not obligatory to administer medications that will only prolong the life of suffering without any chance of cure. Even if the patient is unable to voice his own opinion in this matter, one can consult with immediate members of the family about the patient's wishes had he been able to express them. Such decisions should be made in consultation with a competent Rabbi and the most expert physicians.

Rabbi Feinstein also discusses the topic of the removal of life-support systems from a terminally ill patient[49]. A respirator or other life support instrument may only be removed if it has been definitively established that the patient is dead by Jewish legal criteria, including the absence of spontaneous respiration. If the intravenous injection of a radioactive isotope shows no circulation to the brain including the brain stem, the patient can be considered to be physiologically decapitated, and if all other signs of death are present (e.g., no reflexes, absent caloric responses, flat electroencephalogram, etc.), the respirator may be removed.

Summary and Conclusions

Judaism considers a human life to have infinite value. Therefore, physicians and other health care givers are obligated to heal the sick and prolong life. Physicians are not only given divine license to practice medicine but are also mandated to use their skills to heal the sick. Failure or refusal to do so with resultant negative impact on the patient constitutes a transgression on the part of the physician.

Patients are also duty bound to seek healing from a physician when they are ill and not rely on divine intervention or faith healing. Patients are charged with preserving their health and restoring it when ailing in order to be able to serve the Lord in a state of good health.

The physician's obligation to heal extends even to the care of patients with contagious or communicable diseases if the risk to the physician is small. If the risk is very substantial, physicians are not obligated to endanger their own lives. During plague epidemics, those who cared for patients were highly paid for their perilous work.

Jewish law requires physicians to do everything in their power to prolong life, but prohibits the use of measures that prolong the act of dying. To save a life, all Jewish religious laws are automatically suspended, the only exceptions being idolatry, forbidden sexual relations and murder. In Jewish law and moral teaching, "the value of human life is infinite and beyond measure, so that any part of life - even if only an hour or a second - is of precisely the same worth as seventy years of it, just as any fraction of infinity, being indivisible, remains infinite[50]."

Jewish teaching proclaims the sanctity of human life. The physician is given divine license to heal, but not to hasten death. Every human being is morally expected to help another human in distress including a dying patient. The physician, family, friends, nurses, social workers and other individuals close to the dying patient are all obligated to provide support, including psychosocial and emotional care, until the very end. Fluids and nutrition are part and parcel of that supportive care, no different from walking, turning, talking, singing, reading or just listening to the dying patient. There are times when specific medical and/or surgical therapies are no longer indicated, appropriate or desirable for a terminal, irreversibly ill dying patient. There is no time, however, when general supportive measures can be abandoned, thereby hastening the patient's demise.

May the One and only true Healer of the sick effect a complete healing of all people suffering from a variety of diseases and illnesses through the hands of His messengers on earth, the human physicians. May the Lord cure all sickness from the face of the earth and may He send us the Messiah and rebuild the Holy Temple in Jerusalem, speedily in our days, Amen.

References*

[1]Exodus 15:26.

[2]Proverbs 3:8.

[3]*Ibid*. 4:22.

[4]Exodus 21:19.

[5]*Baba Kamma* 82a.

[6]Deuteronomy 22:2.

[7]Maimonides, M. *Mishnah Commentary* on Nedarim 4:4.

[8]Leviticus 19:16.

[9]*Sanhedrin* 73a.

[10]Maimonides, M. *Mishneh Torah, Hilchot Rotze'ach* 1:14.

[11]Karo J. *Shulchan Aruch, Yoreh Deah* 336.

[12]Maimonides, M. *Mishneh Torah, Hilchot Deot* 3:3.

[13]*Ibid*. 4:23.

[14]*Sanhedrin* 17b.

[15]Maimonides, M. *Mishneh Torah, Hilchot Deot* 4:1.

[16]*Baba Kamma* 46b.

[17]*Yoma* 83b.

[18]*Abodah Zarah* 28b.

[19]*Baba Metzia* 85b.

[20]*Baba Kamma* 85a.

[21]Maimonides, M. *Mishneh Torah, Hilchot Rotze'ach* 1:14.

[22]Karo, J. *Shulchan Aruch, Choshen Mishpat* 426:1.

[23]Karo, J. *Shulchan Aruch, Orach Chayim* 329:8.

[24]Yerushalmi *Terumot*, end of chapter 8, according to *Ha'amek She'elah, She'iltot* 14.

[25]*Sanhedrin* 73a, according to *Agudat Aizov, Derushim* folio 3b and *Hashmatot* folio 38b.

[26]Zimra, D.   Responsa *Radvaz*, Part 5 (Part 2 in *Leshonot HaRambam*, section 1, 582); Responsa *Radvaz*, Part 3, #627, and *Sheiltot Radvaz* 1:52.

[27]Leviticus 19:16.

[28]Feinstein, M. Responsa *Iggrot Moshe, Yoreh Deah*, Part 2, #174:4.

[29]Waldenberg, E.Y. Responsa *Tzitz Eliezer*, Vol. 10, #25:7.

[30]Zuger, A; Miles, S.H. Physicians, AIDS, and occupational risk. Historic traditions and ethical obligations. *J.A.M.A.* 1987; *258*:1924-1928.

[31]Council on Ethical and Judicial Affairs. Ethical issues involved in the growing AIDS crisis. *J.A.M.A.* 1988; *259*:1360-1361.

[32]Health and Policy Committee, American College of Physicians, and the Infectious Diseases Society of America.   The acquired immuno-deficiency syndrome (AIDS) and infection with the human immuno-deficiency virus (HIV). *Ann Int Med* 1988; *108*:460-469.

[33]Professional Responsibility in Treating AIDS Patients. Statement of the Association of American Medical Colleges. *J Med Ed* 1988; *63*:587-590.

[34]Annas, G.J. Not saints, but healers. The legal duties of health care professionals in the AIDS epidemic. *Amer J Public Health* 1988; *78*:844-849.

[35]Emmanuel, E.J. Do physicians have an obligation to treat patients with AIDS? *N Engl J Med* 1988; *318*:1686-1690.

[36]Laskin, D.M. Treatment of patients with AIDS: A Matter of professional ethics. *J Oral Maxillofac Surg* 1988; *46*:719.

[37]Pelligrino, E.D. Altruism, self-interest, and medical ethics. *J.A.M.A.* 1987; *258*:1939-1940.

[38]*Semachot* 1:1.

[39]*Shabbat* 151b.

[40]Waldenberg, E.Y. Responsa *Tzitz Eliezer*, Vol. 5, *Ramat Rachel*, Number 28:5.

[41]*Ibid.* Number 29, and Vol. 10, Number 25:6.

[42]*Ibid.* Vol. 13, Numbers 87 and 89; Vol. 14, Numbers 80 and 81 and Vol. 15, Number 37.

[43]*Ibid.* Vol. 9, Number 46 and Vol. 10, Number 25:4.

[44]Rosner, F. *Modern medicine and Jewish ethics*, Hoboken, NJ and New York, NY, Ktav and Yeshiva University Press 1986, pp. 241-254.

[45]Auerbach, S.Z. *Halachah Urefuah* (M. Hershler, editor). Jerusalem and Chicago, Regensberg Inst., Vol. 2, 1981, p. 131 and pp. 185-190.

[46]Hershler, M. *Halachah Urefuah*, Vol. 2, 1981, pp. 30-52.

[47]Bleich, J.D.   *Judaism and healing*, New York, Ktav, 1981, pp. 134-145.

[48]Feinstein, M.   Responsa *Iggrot Moshe, Choshen Mishpat*, Part 2, Numbers 73, 74 and 75.

[49]Feinstein, M.   Responsa *Iggrot Moshe, Yoreh Deah*, Part 3, Number 132.

[50]Jakobovits, I.   Medical experimentation on humans in Jewish law, in *Jewish bioethics*, ed. by F. Rosner and J.D. Bleich.   New York, Hebrew Publishing Co., 1979, pp. 377-383.

*All talmudic citations are from the Babylonian Talmud unless otherwise stated.

CHAPTER 9

THE JEWISH WAY IN DYING:

THE JEWISH COMPONENT IN HOSPICE CARE

Rabbi Maurice Lamm, D.D.

I nominate two sentences as being freighted with the most tragic overtones known to humanity: "We doctors have done everything we can. Now the patient is in God's hands." These words trigger a hail of emotions, from anger to fear to jealousy to guilt, that tear the innards of those who care but are helpless. From this moment until the advent of death, the terminal patient and the family experience the most painful and critical hours of their lives.

I

Dying is the juncture between time and eternity. It is twilight, *bein ha-shemashot*, as the Rabbis put it - "not day, not night" - when the sun sinks behind the horizon. It is at the end of day that magnificently, the deep colors of day and night mix and swirl, broad strokes on the brush-painted sky. It is like earth's fall season, the twilight for trees, when the leaves burst forth with a palette of colors that blends the greens and yellows of summer and winter. While in nature, twilight squeezes out the most brilliant and memorable of scenes, in human nature, twilight is a gray, bleak mist as it disappears in the onrushing blackness.

Ideally, this human experience of dying should not be so perceived. After the initial trauma of those two sentences, the dying should experience a stillness, a serenity, a coming-together of all of the events of life, a bottom line that makes everything add up, a peace that until now one never knew. No longer the relentless pressure to "make it," the drive to possess more and more. No more reputation to earn; no impossible goals to reach; no petty power to be acquired; no glorious models to imitate; nobody to impress; no more games to play. Now one knows that the goddess of success makes a mockery of sincere striving. The terminal patient finally, too finally, can become detached from everything which is not truly an extension of self. One can love whom one wishes to love; no more ulterior motives. The individual is left with mind and soul and memories and faith and values, and with only real friends and family. It may be the first time that one can afford to live in purity and in total honesty with the private self.

Yet these times may become intolerable - when the ticking of the clock is too loud, when family members are confused, erupting in anger at no one, blabbering incessantly but to no point, pouring sweetness-without-substance over a sick relative; when the patient does not know what to think, what to say, what to do, what is proper. The mind is transfixed by questions without answers: "Why me? What now? Who will take care?"

The individual has no experience in dealing with this matter. Until this generation, people usually died of catastrophic illness, and the end came too quickly to allow for contemplation. That is why, according to *Halakhah* (Jewish law), the definition of dying, *goses*, is a process that takes at most three days. Today, people more likely die from degenerative disease, and the process of dying is often extended for six months and more. Because people spend more time with the dying, they have more time to be frightened; the mystery becomes greater, the emotional complexities more overwhelming. The dying person, like most people, is used to being accompanied by family or friends in every major step of life. Now death will terminate all relationships with everyone. That is the fear - to let go of the offering hands all around and proceed to the precipice of life slowly and alone.

It is not only that individuals have not dealt with this matter in any creative, significant way. The community has not even put the management of dying on its agenda. The Jewish community, which deals successfully with the daytime concerns of youth movements and old-age homes and family services and hospitals, and also with the nighttime concerns of cemetery and free-burial and conferences on grief, does not ever deal with twilight. Yet, dying is the crisis of life. One can die in fulfillment and with meaning; or in misery - filled with hate and jealousy. The confrontation with death is the greatest test of personality and of culture. May we abandon our people at this crossroad?

II

The Jewish philosophy of dying that is the conceptual base of Jewish hospice is informed by three ideas:

1.   **The value of a person derives from each individual being created in the image of God.** The source of human value is different in classical Greek literature from what it is in Jewish law. To Plato, the value of the human being is directly proportional to one's contribution to society. The Greeks espoused the ideal of the Public Man, the opposite of which the Greeks termed *idiotes*, and upon which they frowned severely. They took that idea to its logical extreme and determined the value of the human being by socially utilitarian standards. The old and the infirm, now useless, were consigned to die by exposure.

Counterposed to the Platonic idea is the Jewish concept of human value. The human being's worth derives solely from being created in the image of God. When God created nature, the Bible indicates no specific intention on God's part, and no specific meaning, therefore, was imposed upon nature, simply: "Let us create heaven and earth." God created each individual with a specific pre-condition and clearly-defined purpose: "In God's image." He designated that image as the essential nature of creation. As a consequence of being created in God's image, the human has an integrity and a worth by God-given right, regardless of one's socially utilitarian value. No matter the condition of body or mind - even if one is unconscious or powerless - one retains that inalienable integrity.

In Jewish literature and law, the inherent dignity of the individual is compared to the dignity of the Torah scroll. The death of an individual, for example, is equivalent to the burning of a Torah. In both cases, the onlooker is required to rend his or her garments. As the Torah, used for holy purposes, retains this holiness even when it becomes religiously disqualified, so the human, having been created with the sanctity of God's image, retains dignity even in death, when the image disintegrates. The human remains possess the holiness that characterizes the disqualified Torah scroll itself. Thus, one may not dishonor a corpse, as one may not desecrate the scroll. Surely in dying, even as in death, one retains the integrity of having been created in God's image.

In fact, this Torah view of human worth is the basis of social work. The Western religions, derived philosophically from the Jewish base, hold that all people - especially those who are sick and infirm, or too young to care for themselves - are the subjects of social work practice.

This philosophic attitude translates itself into practical behavioral application in Jewish law. For example, the Torah mandates quick burial because it compares the human being to a king's wayward twin brother who is being hanged. When people pass by, they say: "There hangs the king." The brother's hanging reflects upon the dignity of the king. In much the same way, the rabbis reasoned, if we unnecessarily leave a human corpse to linger unburied, shame accrues to the King of Kings, whose image resides in the human "twin."

2.   **Dying must be confronted as a new reality.** Hans Borkenau divided cultures into death-defying ones, death-accepting ones and death-denying ones.

The Egyptian culture, against which the Israelites rebelled, built society around the glorification of death, symbolized permanently by the pyramids.

Clearly, the American culture is a death-denying one. In an era of possible nuclear destruction, and of the graphic nightly portrayal of bloodshed on television, this is comically absurd. We deny death by diversion, stupefaction, a closing of the eyes, wishful thinking. We repress our fear of death by developing the art of embalming - berouging the dead to make them look alive; by having family sit apart from friends at the mortuary service; and by masking the graves with green mats and consigning the burial to hired diggers. Indeed, we also consign the dying, in turn, to the specialist, the general practitioner, the charge nurse, the private nurse, the rabbi, the convalescent home owner and finally, the mortician. Someone else is always having to handle that terrible reality. "We can't bear to see it," we say in self-indulging compassion.

But by history and theology, Judaism is death-defying. Of all the forms of ritual impurity, the most severe defilement is caused by contact with a dead body. Contrarily, holiness is identified with life. We refer to a "God of Life," and we are unable to accept a "dead god." Through the centuries, the Jew followed the attitude so well expressed by Dylan Thomas - "Rage, rage against the dying of the light" - and our survival relates directly to this attitude.

Not only does Judaism defy death, but, as a consequence of the sin of Adam, it even refuses to consider death a natural phenomenon. It is, as Adin Steinsalz terms it, "the disease of life" (Death Will Be Defeated," *Israel Magazine*, 1969, 2:2, pp. 35-36). Death is a distortion, a perversion of the holiness associated with life. One is to do battle against the "spirit of defilement" which, in fact, is a lifelong battle against death, considered to be the worst defect of this world. The climactic, last phrase of the traditional funeral service is *bila ha-mavet la-netzach*, "May God swallow death forever." In the end, the human will be victorious; death will be defeated. *Herpat amo*, "the 'shame' of His people will He remove from the earth." This is not only a fond wish; it is a mandate to Jews to struggle against the end which inevitably will engulf us all. This philosophy informs the obstinate Jewish refusal to give up on life even against the most insurmountable medical odds. It explains the profound reluctance to pull plugs and stop treatments.

But we must live our daily lives facing the reality that in the end we will die. This realization mandates our confrontation with the process of dying. The traditional Jew was expected to prepare for death. One sewed one's own shrouds, purchased a burial plot while in the blossom of life, left a will, arranged for a funeral and handled one's own death as the necessary, though ever-present evil that it is. One must accept death after defying it to the last. But the repression of the reality of death is an irreligious attitude, and our elaborate attempts at its denial are a religious absurdity.

In this sense, we are called upon to confront the reality of dying. In Jewish law, even such mundane items as contract and will are guided by different standards during these fateful days. It is a new reality, requiring new attitudes. It is not life as usual, and it is not the resignation of death. Hospice is effective to the degree that it looks upon the process of dying as a new stage of existence and uses different norms to realize a person's humanity.

3.   Dying is not primarily a scientific event. Judaism makes a clear distinction between *bios* and *humanum*: physicality and humanity. It is important to determine at which point before birth the fetus goes from *bios* to *humanum*, from a simple, physical organism to a human being; and at dying, at which point the *humanum* returns to *bios*, when a person loses distinctive sanctity as a human being and becomes a vegetating organism. The *Halakhah*, for this reason, extends a person's *humanum* even well beyond the conscious state - until the last breath of existence as a person.

Judaism forcefully and legally affirms that the human being may never be treated solely as *bios*, even during the terminal process of dying. The individual is not primarily a fact. Dying is not primarily a scientific event. It is a human one. During that period, the person has to be treated more humanely, more sensitively, not less, and with greater warmth.

The care given a person is a demonstration of whether the caregiver's emphasis is on *bios* or on *humanum*. Judaism long ago concerned itself not primarily with sickness, but with the sick person. The *Midrash* says that even when there are few moments left to life, we must advise the dying: "Eat this, drink that," even though it cannot make any possible difference. There is a deep concern for the prevention of human pain, which was uppermost in the rabbis' minds, even when dealing with the ordinary pain of healthy people. All religious requirements are exempted in the face of pain. The Hebrew word for doctor, *rofeh*, derives from the Hebrew word *rapeh*, which means to ease or to assuage.

Hospitals, which treat *bios* exclusively, characteristically do not relate to a sense of shame on the part of the patient, to privacy, to personal delicacy or to the need for warmth. The hospice -- which emphasizes the *humanum* component and which treats not only the illness but the patient, by providing a team of psychologists, clergy, social workers, doctors and nurses and mainly, family and volunteers -- has a primary concern for human comfort and for the prevention of pain and its control.

The difference between an emphasis on *bios* or on *humanum* is tellingly illustrated in the style of informing the patient of his or her terminal state. One can declare it in a direct and correct clinical diagnosis. But, with an emphasis on the *humanum*, the telling can be a gradual self-revelation, a sort of Socratic self-understanding. After all, the shortest distance between two points is not necessarily a straight line, when the straight line deals with a personal cataclysm, the upsetting of the whole natural order. If the patient chooses to deny the validity of the medical conclusion, Judaism's attitude is to respect that denial. Helmut Thielicke quotes a Japanese doctor who noted, "There are lies that express profound human love." Truth we should tell, but the superior value is not truth but humanity. In all cases the old folk-wisdom obtains: "Be a *mentsch* (good person)."

The care of the terminally ill, then, must embody these fundamental principles: that people are created in the image of God and retain their integrity no matter who or in what condition they are; that a person's humanity should elicit from us sensitivity and delicacy; that while defying death is an ideality and a hope, the reality of our situation requires that we struggle to preserve life and, failing that, we struggle to preserve humanity, so long as one lives. We were created as human beings; we must nurture that creation by being human.

III

These underlying attitudes of the Jewish religion are expressed in specific strategies that ameliorate the agony of the dying situation.

Judaism must translate its moral axioms into policies of healthy behavior, virtually into a medicine-bag of attitudes which make the twilight meaningful. These attitudes inform the Jewish component in hospice care. The Jewish part deals not only with the *Halakhah* of medical ethics, but with the *Halakhah* of care ethics. As there is a Jewish way of living, there is a Jewish way of dying - and of caring for the dying. The rich Jewish heritage, which through the centuries has experienced each individual in the zenith of growth and the nadir of decline, has designed helping strategies for coping with the problems of the severely ill.

1.   **Loneliness.**   That a dying person is lonely is, of course, understandable. This loneliness is due, in part, to the shock of being thrown back on one's own resources and knowing that the road to one's ultimate destiny will be traveled wholly alone, without any company.

But the dying are lonely for at least two other reasons:

First, they have already begun to mourn their own dying, and the world that will go on without their presence and direction. In Hebrew, the word for mourner is *avel*, which means, "one who withdraws." Not only does the family withdraw, become *avelim*, after a person's death; the patient, too, begins now to withdraw.

Second, the dying are alone not only because of their own psychological state, but because others cause them to suffer the Pariah Syndrome; the patient is placed outside the social pale. If death is a terminus of relationships, then dying is its prelude, and relationships already now begin to become strained and to alter. It is like a candle flame about to be extinguished, that flickers and sputters before it dies. Among the flickerings in personal relationships are the friends and relatives who shy away from the severely ill because they do not know what to say, how to express their genuine feelings of remorse. The caricature drawn by one artist shows a man in a wheelchair and behind him his wife. They are alone in a corner of the room while their friends are in another corner heatedly discussing business. Even close friends express only artificial feelings; they look away, stutter, have no ability to identify, surely to empathize with the patient. The patient becomes amputated from the living body politic. The patient becomes passive, abandoned and disconnected precisely when the need is for connectedness, in order to overcome the forbidding loneliness of one's own dying.

Judaism addresses itself to this problem through the religious requirement of *bikur cholim*, visiting the sick. The sick visitation is not merely a practice of social etiquette, but the fulfillment of a religious obligation.   Unfortunately, the structure and content of this important function are rarely properly focused.   It is simply an exercise in undiscerning sweetness - important, but not crucially helpful. We pay scant attention to what the tradition demands from this religious institution and how psychological findings can enrich it.

Visits should be frequent but of short duration, in keeping with the patient's fatigue threshold. We are not to hover over the bed, not to stand, but to sit on the patient's level. The patient is constantly looking up at doctors and nurses and visitors and made to feel like an object "over" whom people work. We must never leave without praying in the patient's presence. We must never leave without expressing hope.

The very presence of people is a therapeutic presence and considered a very great *mitzvah*. It reassures the patient of continuing worth as an individual and reinforces feelings of being an integral member of the family and the community. Traditionally, in fact, a *minyan* of ten Jews was gathered to be present at the expected moment of life's expiration.

2.   The need for apology. Jewish tradition understood that in order to achieve a degree of inner peace, the patient needs the process of *mehillah*, the asking of forgiveness from those wronged. It is wiping the slate clean, an unburdening of the accumulated baggage of a lifetime. Indeed, there is another form of *mehillah* that the patient needs. Despite the fact that death is not an act of will on the part of the patient, many patients need to apologize, to seek "permission" for leaving their families and for the pain that they cause them by dying. This need may not be expressed openly, and it may require a response of only a look of recognition, a holding of hands; but it should not be mocked or ignored.

3.   Prayer. Maimonides rules that no *bikur cholim* is complete without prayer for the sick.

Prayer is considered a gift, not an obligation; and it can be of great comfort to many patients. There is formal prayer, recited from the prayer book three times daily in the traditional manner. There is also informal prayer, which can be recited in any language, in any posture, at any time. This prayer may ask for an extension of life or for a remission from pain. It may also be used to vent anger and complaint, even to ask for a rapid death. Prayer is especially valuable at this time because it allows for the articulation of hopes and fears in an accepted and elevated manner, and because it is offered as a communication from one who is powerless to the Almighty. Even those who do not customarily pray, or even believe in God, are often moved to do so in such conditions. "Pray for me" is a phrase often heard in hospital corridors. "Pray for yourself" is equally valid and even more helpful.

Curiously, the Code of Jewish Law suggests that prayer in the synagogue or outside the room should be recited in Hebrew. The prayer in the patient's room, however, should be recited in any language that is understandable to the patient. Prayer, in this sense, serves the twofold purpose of petitioning God and of comforting the sick. Also, it is entirely proper and probably very comforting to the patient to recite a prayer for the sick in the synagogue at the open Torah scroll. This prayer is called *mi she-berakh*.

Traditionally, over the centuries, the last syllables uttered by Jews as life nears its end are the words of a confessional prayer, called *Viddui*. It is a cumulative apology for the misdeeds of a lifetime. The sages considered it extremely valuable as an expiation for all sins. It is brief and moving. Great care should be taken in introducing this prayer delicately, assuring the patient that many have recited the prayer and survived. If this prayer might traumatize the patient, it should not be recited. A brief form of confession is as follows:

> *Tehai mitati kapparah al kol avonotai*: I acknowledge unto Thee, O Lord my God and God of my fathers, that both my cure and my death are in Thy hand. May it be Thy will to grant me a perfect healing. Yet if Thou has decreed that I should die, may my death expiate all the sins which I have committed before Thee, and grant me a portion in the Garden of Eden and cause me to merit the life of the World to Come, which is reserved for the righteous. Hear, O Israel, the Lord our God, the Lord is One.

4.   Hope. What hope is possible for the dying? Yet, in the midst of this apparently hopeless situation, one is mandated by the Jewish tradition to inject hope into every visit, every conversation. But what can one hope for? Pessimists are fond of saying that from the moment of birth one

proceeds every day closer to death. Helmut Thielicke notes that this saying
is not quite true. The analogy that he gives is to a person walking. Every
step is a falling and yet at the very last moment, before the person really
falls, he or she stretches forth the other leg and straightens out again. After
a series of fallings and risings, a person finds that progress has been made
through these ups and downs. But dying is, after all, the time of the final
falling. What straightening up may come? What rising sun can be expected
from this twilight? Yet hope we must. One can hope for less pain, for the
future happiness of children, for the family's continuation of the values one
has spent a lifetime instilling.   While there should be an intelligent
awareness of hope's limitation in this situation, a sincere expression of hope
is required by the tradition. In fact, Jews believe that death may be the
beginning of exaltation, a reunion of the divine image with the divine source
of being, as Abraham J. Heschel says:

> Death is not sensed as a defeat but as a summation, an arrival, a
> conclusion. Our ultimate hope has no specific content, our hope is
> God. We trust that He will not desert those that trust in Him. The
> meaning as well as mode of being which man hopes to attain beyond
> the threshold of dying remains an impenetrable mystery, yet it is the
> thought of being in God's knowing that may be both at the root and
> the symbol of the ultimate hope.   ("Reflections On Death,"
> *Conservative Judaism*, Fall, 1973, pp. 3-9)

5.   **Power.** The dying patient finds the self in a passive condition
-- powerless to initiate significant actions or make significant decisions;
tested and turned and injected; cried over and spoken of and prayed for.
One has effectively been removed from the dynamic world. The Jewish
tradition provides for specific activities which give the patient a sense of
power - thoughts to be managed, projects to be executed which can excite
the mind and spark one's imagination to think creatively, even during this
time.

a)   **Ethical Wills.** In order to give initiative to the terminal
patient, one should be encouraged to write an ethical will. This is an
ancient Jewish device. People should leave their families not only an
inheritance, but also a heritage. A parent may not have been able to
communicate effectively with a child or grandchild. This device affords the

patient the opportunity to leave the loved ones a sense of purpose in life, values and beliefs, in a format that will be treasured after death.

b)   Oral History. Another "project" which is of clear value at this time is leaving behind the legacy of an oral history. By speaking into a tape recorder, the patient can give living roots to the family, e.g., details of childhood, education, family relationships, beliefs and dreams. A mate, child or nurse can assist by asking pertinent questions and guiding the conversation. This process invokes good feelings, both in recalling pleasant memories during days of recording the personal history, and then in giving children a gift volume describing their family roots. It is little short of an intimation of immortality.

c)   Charity. The Jewish sages said that "Charity rescues from death." Obviously the sages were not speaking of magic. They meant that it saves the dying from the feeling of death. Distributing charity, no matter who the recipient or what the amount, and deliberating as to who should receive it, may give a person a feeling of strength and a sense of being alive.

d)   "Setting the house in order." The time of dying is a time for arrangements for the family, for the handling of one's own personal attitudes and status and relationships. The Patriarch Jacob was blessed with illness, the rabbis say, in order that he might prepare for death. Isaiah, the Prophet, tells King Hezekiah: "Set thy house in order, for thou shalt die, not live."

6.   Love. Since time is now limited, life becomes ever more precious, and the relationship between the family and the dying person should be intensified in depth and quality. It should be a period when loved ones sustain and cherish the patient. It may be that the relationship was strained for many years, that there were many dissonances, even much bickering, and that therefore the expression of love now suddenly demonstrated is felt to be a hypocrisy. But now life is new and love can begin anew. Rabbi Eliyahu Dessler, one of this century's greatest Jewish ethicists, asks: which comes first - giving or loving? The common answer is that one gives to a person whom one already loves. The reverse is also true. One loves the person to whom one has given. The more parents give to a child who is in need, the more the love grows.

At a time of terminal illness, the family should give of themselves. They should hug and stroke and touch the patient. The giving may exalt love to a level that was hitherto unimaginable.

The art of loving is most strained when you love someone who is approaching death. Done properly, love can rise to its most intense level at precisely this moment; feelings can become more authentic than at any other time in life; the capacity for giving and for sheer goodness can be unimaginable; and the effect can physically lengthen a person's life and make the last moments beautiful. These last expressions of love plumb our deepest personal resources.

A friend of mine, Jack, was trying to impel his wife, Mary, to take more medicine in her dying days. He said to her, "Mary, I'm not giving you poison." Mary looked at him and said, "Jack, I never thought you were capable of caring for me so much. Even if you gave me poison, from you I would take it as medicine."

It is twilight. As the sun falls behind the horizon, human life, like nature, can produce a burst of color - the color of meaningfulness, of hope and love.

PART III

CLINICAL ISSUES

CHAPTER 10

ETHICAL DILEMMAS IN MEDICAL PRACTICE

Fred Rosner, M.D.

Medical practitioners are today faced with a host of ethical, moral, legal and psychosocial issues in the care of their patients, over and above the standard medical considerations. This essay discusses some of these ethical dilemmas, specifically those relating to patients' rights, the care of the terminally ill, the allocation of scarce medical resources and informed consent.

PATIENTS' RIGHTS

Among patient rights are the right to know the truth, the right to treatment, the right to refuse treatment and the right not to be resuscitated. None of these are absolute rights, however.

The Right to Know

Although a person has a right to know that he has a very serious and even fatal disease, the physician may occasionally withhold such information if the patient might be harmed by having such knowledge. A person who would attempt suicide upon learning that he has a fatal illness should probably not be told. Ordinarily, however, a physician should not lie to a patient about the diagnosis or prognosis of the illness just to save the patient some anxiety and grief.

What if the family asks the doctor to withhold the information from the patient? Ordinarily the family has no right to control disclosure of information unless such disclosure would produce mental anguish (Hebrew: *tiruf hada' at*). What if the patient asks the doctor to withhold information about the diagnosis and prognosis from the family? Here, the physician-patient confidentiality relationship may allow or even require the doctor not to disclose the information to the family.

Once the decision to inform the patient about his condition and outlook has been made, it is important to know how, when and where the information should be disclosed, who should do the disclosing and what should be said. If a patient is to be told about incurable cancer, it should be done with compassion and humaneness, in a comfortable private environment and only after a firm doctor-patient relationship has been established, not at the first visit. Most often the physician discloses the information, but occasionally a family member, clergyman or even medical student may be the best person to disclose the information to the patient. The best possible outcome should be portrayed, always leaving room for hope. Assurance of pain relief and comfort provision and psychosocial support to the very end must be communicated to the patient as part of the disclosure: "We will be with you all the way. We hope you will be among the patients who respond well to the anticancer treatment. Many patients with cancer are cured. We hope you will be one of them, etc."

The Right to Treatment

All patients should have access to medical care as a right. However, a patient cannot always select his own physician. Patients in public hospitals are assigned one or more physicians to provide for their care. The family has no right to ask that treatment be stopped on a patient who wishes such treatment to be continued.

How far does the patient's right to treatment extend? Does every person with end-stage heart disease or liver disease have a right to a heart or a liver transplant, respectively, at a cost of approximately a quarter of a million dollars each? Society cannot afford to provide everything for everybody. Does a patient have a right to determine the extent and type of medical care that he is to receive? Does a patient have a right to receive palliative care if he has rejected diagnostic work-up and specific life-saving care? Does a critically ill patient have the right to determine which drugs will be used in his treatment?

The Right to Refuse Treatment

The patient has the legal right in Western society to refuse diagnostic work-up and medical treatment that would prolong his life. What if the doctors disagree with the patient's choice to refuse medical care? When is a patient competent to refuse medical care? Who determines competency? What should doctors do when they are uncertain about the patient's competency when he refuses treatment? What happens if a doctor treats a competent patient against his wishes in order to keep him alive? Do family members or surrogates have a right to refuse treatment on behalf of a patient who does not have the capacity to decide for himself?

The Right Not to Be Resuscitated

In 1988 New York State passed a law which requires that all patients who may have a cardiorespiratory arrest be asked by their physicians whether or not they wish to be resuscitated in such an eventuality. The intent of the law was to assure the patient his right not to be resuscitated. Unless a written order not to resuscitate is entered into the patient's medical record, every patient is presumed to wish resuscitative efforts and these must be applied even if the patient has an irreversible, incurable condition such as terminal, widespread metastatic cancer. Thus, legal attempts to assure patient's rights are interfering with the proper practice of medicine and are coercing medical staff to apply cardiopulmonary resuscitation where it is not appropriate.

Writing in the *Wall Street Journal* (March 9, 1989), Dr. Kenneth Prager stated that it has become increasingly difficult to die in a New York hospital without first being subjected to cardiopulmonary resuscitation (CPR), due to a state law that went into effect last April. Under the banners of patients' rights and combating physician "paternalism," the State Department of Health dealt a blow to good medical care by dictating the manner in which physicians may withhold CPR from patients in all state health-care facilities. It was left to the discretion of the patient's physician to determine the suitability of CPR. The patient was given the benefit of any conceivable doubt. A decision was reached only after careful consideration of the patient's medical condition and following discussion, when appropriate, with the patient and his relatives, friends and clergy.

Physicians now have no choice but to discuss with every patient who might need CPR whether to carry out this procedure. This is not as simple as it sounds. Critically ill patients often cannot cope with the stress of discussing the possibility of their imminent death and of rationally weighing the pros and cons of CPR. They often have no idea of what the procedure involves and of the possible state to which they might be restored in the event of a "successful" resuscitation. To some patients, the mere discussion of these issues implies a weakening of their physician's resolve to help them.

When a patient is not emotionally or mentally competent to discuss these issues, the task falls to a "surrogate," who usually is the next of kin. If a do-not-resuscitate (DNR) order is decided upon, the surrogate must sign the document that officially withholds CPR from the dying patient. No matter how appropriate the decision, the act of signing a legal document that symbolically finalizes their beloved's death is something that many people cannot do. The order is not signed, and another futile CPR is carried out. Family disagreements or unreachable surrogates may also lead to a decision that is not in the patient's best interest.

Prager concluded by saying that the New York State DNR law demonstrates how indiscriminate advocacy of patients' rights can confuse the appropriate arena for physician judgment with "paternalism" and can lead to unfortunate results. Let the rest of the nation take note: "For many of New York's terminally ill, the road to eternal rest has been paved with useless and mischievous obstacles created by good intentions."

PATIENTS' MORAL OBLIGATIONS

Although patients have the legal right to know their diagnosis and prognosis, the legal right to treatment and to refuse treatment, and the legal right not to be resuscitated, patients also have moral obligations to seek healing when they are sick, to care for their bodies which are given to them "on loan" by God and over which they serve as stewards, to accept standard medical workup and therapy for their illness, to be guided by the advice of their physicians and to be healthy, productive members of society.

The extreme swing from paternalism two and three decades ago, when doctors made all the decisions without always consulting the patient, to the present patient-autonomy approach, in which the patient makes all the decisions, notwithstanding the doctor's recommendations, represents a shift from one extreme to another.

The right to know and the right to treatment have now been extended to the point where they are equated with the right to decide. The patient now is not only involved in decision-making but often makes the decision because of the right to autonomy. When a woman presents to the doctor with a lump in her breast which on biopsy is proven to be malignant, the physician nowadays has to present the patient with a menu of therapeutic options from which to choose: Madam, would you like a lumpectomy or simple mastectomy or radical mastectomy or modified radical mastectomy? Would you like post-operative radiation or no post-operative radiation? Would you like adjuvant chemotherapy or no adjuvant chemotherapy?

Of course, certain rights are not open to much discussion or dispute. Smokers, for example, have the right to lung cancer, the right to heart disease, the right to emphysema, the right to bladder cancer, etc. On the other hand, smokers also have the moral obligation to avoid all these ills and to preserve their health by abandoning this pernicious habit or addiction.

THE LIVING WILL: HELP OR HINDRANCE

The common theme of living wills or natural death statutes is the endorsement of the right of a competent patient to sign a binding directive refusing life-prolonging measures during terminal illness. I will not even attempt to define "competent" since that term usually implies a legal rather than medical connotation. But what does "life-prolonging" mean? How prolonged? One minute, one hour, one day, one week? If the value of human life is infinite, as I believe it is, one second or one hour of life is of precisely the same worth as months or years of it, just as any fraction of infinity, being indivisible, remains infinite. What is the difference between life-prolonging and death-prolonging? How does one draw the distinction?

What does the phrase "terminal illness" mean? How terminal? One hour, one day, one week? A small but significant fraction of patients pronounced terminally ill by their attending physicians survive for a much longer period of time than predicted, as exemplified by Karen Quinlan who lived many years after her respirator was withdrawn. Many living wills incorporate the terms "permanent," "irreversible," "imminently dying," "chronic vegetative state," to which one can ask: How permanent? How irreversible? How imminent? How chronic?

Another confusing catch phrase is "heroic or extraordinary measures to prolong life." Is the use of a respirator heroic or extraordinary? How about a blood transfusion? Antibiotics? Intravenous fluids? A feeding tube? Analgesics? Where does one draw the line? Even if one accepts the use of antibiotics as standard therapy for pneumonia in you or me, would such treatment be heroic or extraordinary in a dying cancer patient? I think not. The use of cardiac monitors for patients admitted to intensive care units with precordial chest pain is standard practice today. Yet only a decade ago, such monitors were scarce, expensive and infrequently used. Thus, what is standard practice today was heroic or extraordinary only a decade ago. In many cases, extraordinary therapy may restore critically ill or even unconscious patients to a functional life.

Although the living will is an expression of the patient's autonomy, such a written document can be as much a hindrance as a help to the physicians and family faced with carrying out the wishes cited therein. Because of the lack of specificity and uncertainty of prognosis, the provisions of the living will may be activated prematurely. The existence of the will might deprive the patient of the full concern of the medical team who may not exert the maximal effort demanded by the patient's condition. During the five-year period when the living will is usually in effect, the patient may change his mind but not formally rescind the declaration.

The legally-sanctioned living will presumes that the patient has a right to prematurely terminate his life and to impose ethical value judgments upon physicians and other members of the medical team who are instructed to assist the patient in this hastening of death under the terms of the will. Does not a living will contradict society's declared obligation to preserve and protect the health and life of its citizens? From the moral viewpoint, the living will denies the preciousness and infinite value of human life. Here is where the "slippery slope" begins.

DECISION-MAKING IN AN INTENSIVE CARE UNIT

Most intensive care units have limited capacity. Hence, medical and ethical decisions have to be made in regard to which patients gain admission to the ICU and which are denied such admission because of a scarcity of beds or because of inappropriateness for that patient to be in an ICU. Generally, the following questions are asked in regard to admitting a patient to an ICU: Is the disease process irreversible? Is the condition terminal? Is the disease incurable? Discharging a patient from the ICU to make room for another patient often depends on answers to the following questions: Is intensive care appropriate for the patient? Is it doing any good? Should it be stopped?

The decisions used to be made solely by the physician. That was the era of paternalism. Nowadays, the patient, family and others participate. The extent of the decision or what is decided is also important. Should the patient receive total therapy, total therapy but no cardiopulmonary resuscitation, "normal" therapy but no extraordinary measures, only supportive care but no medical interventions? The decisions are made through communication, discussion, reasoning and sometimes even bargaining.

Arguments for the withdrawal of therapy in an ICU setting include patient autonomy (i.e., the patient refuses further therapy), triage (e.g., the ICU is full and a "salvageable" patient is waiting for an ICU bed), economic factors (i.e., it is too expensive to keep the patient in the ICU), brain death, chronic persistent vegetative state, quality of life (e.g., deep coma), medical judgment (e.g., the physicians feel therapy is no longer appropriate) and burdens on the patient exceeding the benefits.

ALLOCATION OF SCARCE MEDICAL RESOURCES

Examples of medical decision-making in the presence of scarcity include the following: If there is only one dialysis machine but three patients need dialysis, who gets it? If there is one intensive care bed available but two patients need it, who gets it?

Allocation decisions are often made in a two-step process whereby one first excludes certain patients from receiving the therapy and then one selects from the remaining patients who is to receive the treatment. In the classic hemodialysis situation, factors of exclusion may include age, disease, ability to pay, social worth of the individual, bias, treatment requirements (e.g., need for running water and electricity for home dialysis), hospital orientation (e.g., veterans' hospitals exclude non-veterans), and patient desires (e.g., patient's preference for a particular physician). After these exclusionary criteria have been applied, patients are selected from the remaining pool on the basis of life expectancy, family role, contributions to society, prospect of success and other criteria.

All these exclusion and selection criteria can be criticized on moral and ethical grounds. Only a first-come, first-served approach seems to be totally equitable. However, some exceptions may have to be made for pragmatic reasons. Should a brilliant scientist receive preference in the allocation of a scarce resource over an unemployed alcoholic? Should a mother of six children be dialyzed in preference to a drug addict? Practical necessity and the public conscience may require exceptions to be made.

The above allocation decisions are made by physicians and hospitals. There are also allocation decisions made by the government or society at large. Should the government develop a new bomber or build another aircraft carrier for the defense of the country or should these financial resources be allocated to the health of its citizens? How should the limited dollars available for health be allocated? Should hemodialysis take priority over hypertension screening or well-baby clinics or cancer research? Political decisions about the allocation of health dollars are often based on considerations other than rational medical thinking.

The governmental macro-allocation process differs in several respects from the micro-allocation decisions of the physician at the bedside. The macro-allocation process is far removed from the clinical setting, is impersonal and not emotionally charged, involves large numbers of people on a national scale, and is not subject to the urgency of acting swiftly in a life or death situation.

In an article on the availability of organ transplantation in the July 5, 1984 issue of the *New England Journal of Medicine*, the questionnaire asked, "Does liver or heart transplantation offer a proper way of using our resources, given other available areas of investment?   Is there moral authority to use state force to redistribute financial resources so as to provide transplantations for all who would benefit from the procedure? How ought one fairly to resolve controversies in this area when there is important moral disagreement?" The February 2, 1984 issue of the *Journal* presents ethical issues in the implantation of the total artificial heart, including financial considerations, risk-to-benefit ratio, selection criteria, quality of life, and informed consent.

INFORMED CONSENT

The legal basis for informed consent was enunciated by Judge Benjamin Cardozo in 1914 as follows:

Every human being of adult years and sound mind has a right to determine what shall be done with his own body, and a surgeon who performs an operation without his patient's consent commits an assault for which he is liable in damages.

Consent can be expressed by the patient either orally or in writing, or consent can be implied and understood by reasonable inference from the conduct of the patient. If the patient voluntarily undresses to allow the doctor to examine him/her, consent for the physical examination is implied by the act of removing one's clothes. If the patient stretches forth his arm to allow the physician to draw a sample of blood, consent is implied.

In the United States, consent must be "informed" which means that the patient understands the procedure to which he or she is consenting and the potential risks and benefits involved. Prior to 1970 the "professional community" standard required the physician to disclose to the patient that which responsible practitioners in the same or similar situations would disclose. Since 1970, the "reasonable patient" standard of informed consent focuses on the informational needs of an average, reasonable patient rather than on professionally established standards of disclosure. The information to be provided by the physician includes the diagnosis (i.e., the patient's condition or problem), the nature and purpose of the proposed treatment, the probability that the proposed treatment will be successful, feasible treatment alternatives, and the prognosis if the proposed treatment is not given.

There are exceptions to the legal requirements of informed consent. These include medical emergencies, therapeutic privilege where disclosure might harm the patient, waivers whereby the patient waives the right to be informed and/or to consent, and incompetency.

The ethical foundations for informed consent are the maximization of good to the patient, the minimization of harm to the patient, a person's right to self-determination (i.e., autonomy) and the maximization of good to society (i.e., utilitarianism).

The opponents of informed consent characterize fully-informed consent as a fairy tale, fiction, a myth, bad medicine, an illusion, a farce, "hazardous to one's health," unbearable, etc.   There are obviously circumstances where full disclosure might be detrimental to the patient and therefore medically contraindicated. Full disclosure of potential risks is not considered appropriate when it might unduly worry a patient and even persuade him or her not to accept treatment deemed to be necessary and beneficial. Some patients don't want to know everything and denial is an important defense mechanism in serious illness. Different physicians have varying views about what should be told to patients about risks of treatment and side effects and what patients and the public think they should be told. Nowadays, the physician should recognize that the patient is entitled to be given adequate information to evaluate whether he or she wishes to accept the benefits and risks of a particular treatment. It is also important for the physician to pay attention not only to what should be told but to who should do the telling, where it should be told, when it should be told, and how it should be told. The manner and timing of disclosure to the patient and the support and comfort of the physician are vital elements in obtaining informed consent for treatment.

Informed consent for medical research is a related but separate topic beyond the scope of this presentation.

CONCLUSION

In this era of diagnosis related groups (DRGs), professional review organizations, cost containment, quality assurance, utilization review, brain death, withholding and/or withdrawing fluids and nutrition from the terminally ill, organ transplantation, in vitro fertilization, embryo transfers, prenatal diagnosis, in utero surgery, and so much more, the practicing physician may become overwhelmed with the numerous ethical, moral, legal and psychosocial issues involved. This essay addresses several medical ethical issues: patients' rights (and obligations), the living will, decision-making in an intensive care unit, the allocation of scarce medical resources, and informed consent. Some of the pitfalls and difficulties associated with these topics are pointed out.

CHAPTER 11

CARE OF THE TERMINALLY ILL

Rabbi J. David Bleich, Ph.D.

Part I: Physicians' Issues

Although I have a filing cabinet devoted to matters concerning bioethics that contains more folders than I can count, I don't have a folder that carries on it the title "Terminally Ill." The title itself implies a certain mind-set that is well-nigh alien to my way of thinking. To be sure, there are many problems in the treatment of the terminally ill, and many ethical issues that have to be analyzed from a Jewish perspective, but those issues are hardly unique to the care of the terminally ill. But that should not be terribly surprising. The great repository of Jewish teaching and Jewish tradition, the *Shulhan Arukh* -- the Code of Jewish Law -- contains but one brief section embodying no more than a few short paragraphs dealing with the treatment of the terminally ill.

Let me try to begin from the beginning by saying that in order to place these issues in proper perspective it is necessary to be aware of the fact that, in Judaism, there exists a certain theological tension with regard to the practice of medicine in general. One of the early Karaite heresies was the denial of the legitimacy of medicine *in toto*. The Karaites even managed to cite a biblical verse in support of their position -- "*ki ani ha-*

Shem rofe'kha" -- "for I the Lord am your physician" (Exodus 15:26); and if God is the physician, who needs a second opinion? Certainly if one recognizes, as Judaism does, that God exercises providential guardianship over the universe and that reward and punishment are meted out in accordance with a person's deeds, the problem becomes a formidable one. If God Himself visits sickness and affliction upon a human being, how dare mortal man interfere with physiological processes in an attempt to reverse the course of disease? If, as Judaism does, one accepts the notion of divine providence, the practice of medicine becomes problematic, to say the least. Indeed, if one examines the classic statement in the Mishnah, *Sanhedrin* 73a, regarding the obligation of preserving human life and the obligation to come to the assistance of another individual whose life is in danger -- obligations that are predicated upon the biblical admonition "*lo ta'amod al dam re'ekha"* -- "nor shall you stand idly by the blood of your fellow" (Leviticus 19:16), one finds that the examples given are nontherapeutic in nature. The examples that are given include a person who has fallen into a river and cannot swim to safety, or an individual who is being mauled by a wild animal and a person who is the victim of armed brigands.

It is only in an entirely different Talmudic discussion that there occurs a reference to preservation of the lives of the dangerously ill. The scriptural source of that obligation is a verse ostensibly dealing with liability for tort damages. In addition to compensation that must be made for other damages, Scripture declares "and he shall cause him to be thoroughly healed" (Exodus 21:20); i.e., the tortfeasor must pay any expenses incurred for any medical treatment required as a result of his battery. The Talmud comments "*Mi-ka'an she-nitnah reshut le-rofeh le-rape'ot"* --"from here it is derived that the physician is given permission to heal." Nahmanides, in citing this dictum in his *Torat ha-Adam* declares, "*Hai reshut, reshut de-mitzvah hi.*" The thrust of that dictum is that this verse serves not simply to grant permission to proffer medical treatment, but also to establish an absolute obligation to practice the healing arts. Indeed, the Hebrew term *"reshut,"* as used in this context, should not be understood as meaning "permission" at all, but should be understood as meaning "authority." The Bible gives the physician authority to practice the healing arts, but once that authority has been bestowed upon man, activity pursuant to that authority becomes obligatory because it is subsumed under the general obligation to preserve human life. That notion is incorporated in the extremely precise language in which the obligation is couched in its codification in the

Shulhan Arukh, Yoreh De'ah 336:1.   The *Shulhan Arukh* states very succinctly:

> The Torah gave permission to the physician to heal; moreover, this is a religious precept and is included in the category of saving life; and if the physician withholds his services, it is considered as shedding blood.

In granting the physician the right to practice, the physician is co-opted as an active partner by the Deity in exercising providential guardianship over mortal man. *"Ani El Shaddai"* -- "I am God *Shaddai"* is an expression repeated numerous times in the Bible.   The sages of the Midrash understood the word "Shaddai" to be an acronym, viz., *"Ani she-amarti le-shamayim ve-aretz*: *'Di.'"* "I," said the Creator, "Am the Being who said to heaven and earth: 'Enough'" (*Bereishit Rabbah* 8:7).   God could have chosen to create a universe in which man sustains himself on bread produced by a "breadfruit" tree. It did not have to be the case that the development and maturation of kernels of wheat is arrested so that man must harvest the wheat, grind the tiny kernels of wheat into flour, mix the flour with water, knead the dough and then bake bread. The universe did not have to be designed so that it is necessary for man to harvest cotton or flax, spin thread, weave cloth and then sew a garment. The world could have been created in a manner such that those plants would have continued their developmental process to the point that bread would grow in the field; He could have created a world in which jackets and dresses would grow in fields of flax and cotton. But God determined that man must become an active partner in the process of creation and must bring the divine handiwork to perfection. Similarly, insofar as providential guardianship of man is concerned, God ordained that man become an active partner in that guardianship as well. And so, it turns out that, from the perspective of Judaism, a physician requires not only a diploma from medical school and a license bestowed by a board of examiners, but that he requires divine dispensation as well.

Since the physician requires a divine license, it should not be at all surprising that the license is accompanied by conditions and stipulations, some of them negative, others positive in nature.   Our society licenses physicians but places restrictions upon their activity.   There are certain things a physician might like to be able to do, but he cannot do them because the law forbids him from so doing. He cannot administer a drug that has not been approved by the FDA. There are other things he might prefer not to do, but must do anyway. To maintain his credentials, he must participate in programs of continuing education. To retain a hospital affiliation, he may be required to provide his services *pro bono* in a clinic for a certain number of hours per week or per month. Similarly, insofar as divine dispensation is concerned, it should not be too surprising to find that there are both "thou shalt nots" and "thou shalts" associated with the practice of medicine. Part of the ongoing positive obligation of the physician is the recognition that he is a divine messenger and that, as such, is charged with acting in a manner consistent with the divine mandate. He is charged with being a Good Samaritan. Once the license to practice the healing arts has been granted, he is required to use it in preserving life granted by the Creator.

Thus, the practice of medicine is no different from any other aspect of human behavior designed to rescue human life -- and I made that statement advisedly. To go back to the paradigms presented in the Mishnah in *Sanhedrin*: if an individual is drowning in the river, a Jew is obligated to jump into the water, if it is within his power to do so, and to rescue the accident victim who cannot swim. Certainly, it would be inappropriate for the would-be rescuer, before jumping into the water, to ask questions with regard to the longevity anticipation of the potential drowning victim. Whether the drowning victim is a young child with his or her life yet unfolding, or whether the victim is an octogenarian whose life anticipation is minimal at best, is totally irrelevant with regard to whether the drowning victim should be saved. Similarly, the obligations imposed upon a physician are not limited to restoring an individual to good health, but also include the obligation to prolong life even when a cure is not available. That, after all, is part and parcel of the Jewish view with regard to the sanctity of life. Judaism teaches not simply that every human life is of infinite value, but that every moment of human life is of infinite value.

When the Sages told us "Against your will you live and against your will you die" (*Avot* 4:29) they meant that very literally. Not only is man born and does man die against his will in the sense that a child is born screaming when he comes into this world and later protests when he is called upon to depart from this world, but there are also times when an individual's life is prolonged despite the fact that we recognize very well that he would much prefer to be allowed to slip away peacefully into death's welcoming embrace. Life may have become more of a burden than a person wishes to endure. But, nevertheless, in many, and probably in most cases, there is an obligation to recognize that life must be preserved and that this, too, is part of the Divine mandate.

In order to understand why that is the case and the framework in which this must be understood, let me draw your attention to one of the greatest of Western thinkers, a Greek philosopher by the name of Plato, who, at times, had an uncanny way of presenting authentic Jewish teaching in a very eloquent manner. In this case, he makes the point as eloquently as any Jewish thinker could possibly express it. The scene comes from one of the Platonic dialogues, the *Phadeo*, and depicts the last hours of the life of Socrates. Socrates was about to be executed, unjustly in his opinion, by his fellow Athenians. Socrates' disciples had managed to bribe the warden and they were admitted to his prison cell in order to be in Socrates' company during his last hours. They expected Socrates to be melancholy and despondent. Instead, they entered his cell to find that he was exuberant; Socrates was overcome with happiness. The students, in effect, asked him the question of King Solomon, "*U-le-simhah mah zo osah?*" (Ecclesiastes 2:2) -- "What is the meaning of this jubilation?" Socrates responded by saying in effect, "Why shouldn't I be happy? I'm about to enter upon a much better kind of existence." Moreover, "I've been waiting all my life to die and now at long last it's about to happen." His students responded by asking a follow-up question: "If that is the case, Socrates, then why did you wait for the Athenians? Why didn't you take matters into your own hands at a much younger age and simply commit suicide?" Rather than answering the question, Socrates responded in a typically Semitic way by asking a question of his own. He turned to his students and said, "And what would you think of a cow that does away with itself?" The students replied by saying, "But, of course, that would be immoral -- it's unjust. The master is entitled to the enjoyment of his property and if the cow destroys itself, it is interfering in this proprietor-property relationship. That is theft, it is immoral." To which Socrates responded by saying, "Don't you see that this is exactly the same case. Just as you recognize that a cow cannot interfere in the property-proprietor relationship, don't you also realize that man is the chattel of the gods and that man has no right to intervene in the Creator-creature relationship." Man has no right to do away with himself. Man is

created by God and must wait for the Creator to reclaim the life with which
He has imbued the human organism.

In struggling with biomedical issues, it is important to recognize that
man does not have a proprietary interest in either his life or his body. If
one looks for a legal category in order to explain man's rights and
obligations with regard to his life, and his person, it would be quite accurate
to say that human life is a bailment, that man is a bailee, and that the
Creator is the bailor. God has created man and has entrusted him with this
precious treasure called human life. Life has been entrusted to man for
guardianship and safekeeping. Man is required to preserve and to prolong
that life until such time as God chooses to reclaim it. That does not mean
that this is an easy task. It does not mean that the charge may not be
burdensome. It certainly does not mean that man, left to his own desires,
to his own intelligence and his own very human emotions, might not often
wish otherwise. Indeed, in situations that are unfortunately all too frequent,
it would be only human for a person to wish otherwise.

Even the desire for active termination of human life is no less than
human. One of the mid-19th-century commentaries on the Bible, in
discussing the verse in Genesis that prohibits the taking of the life of a
fellow human being, points to a certain redundancy in the formulation of
that admonition: "But the blood of your lives will I require ... even at the
hands of a man's brother will I require the life of man." (Genesis 9:15).
The concluding phrase of that verse is superfluous. If homicide is a capital
crime it surely follows, *a fortiori*, that fratricide is also a capital crime.
Remarking on this apparent redundancy, *Ha-Ketav ve-ha-Kabbalah* remarks
that ordinarily the taking of a human life is an act of aggression, a
malevolent act that would be condemned by any civilized person. But there
are occasions when the taking of a life is actually an act of kindness, an act
of love; there are occasions when the taking of a life is an act of brotherly
love, when it is an expression of the type of fraternal caring a person would
manifest for his own brother. There are times when human life appears to
be unbearable and it seems to be an act of mercy and compassion to enable
an individual shouldering such a burden to die. Scripture equates such an
act with the taking of human life under the most reprehensible of
circumstances.

There are circumstances in which a patient is afflicted with a terminal illness and -- to use the phrase which is now very much in vogue -- one would very much want to allow that person to die with dignity, yet there is an overriding obligation that not only prevents the physician from assisting that person in terminating his life, but also prevents the physician from passively allowing the patient to slip away quietly and peacefully by requiring active intervention in order to prolong that life. Judaism accepts the notion of man as a *shomer*, as a bailee, who bears a divinely imposed obligation with regard to preservation of life. To be sure, there are times when man would wish to be relieved of that obligation. But so long as the obligation is not removed from him, he dare not shirk it.

I would like to draw your attention to the very eloquent statement of Rabbenu Nissim in his commentary on Tractate *Nedarim* 40a, in which he discusses a Talmudic anecdote regarding a servant of Rabbi Judah the Prince, a woman who was regarded by the Sages of the Talmud as an exemplary personality in her own right. Rabbi Judah was afflicted with a terminal gastrointestinal illness that caused him great suffering. She begged Rabbi Judah's students to desist from their prayers on his behalf. They refused to do so. Rabbenu Nissim, in explaining her request, states that an individual performing the *mitzvah* (commandment) of visiting the sick is required not simply to engage in social chitchat, but to perform some positive service on behalf of the patient. But, queries Rabbenu Nissim, what can you give, what can you do for someone who already has the best possible medical or nursing care? He answers that there is one thing that every patient needs, there is one thing of which a patient can never have too much, and that is prayer. One can always pray for the patient. But, he proceeds to ask, what if one is confronted by a patient whose life has become too burdensome? What can one do for that patient? Rabbenu Nissim answers very succinctly that, to be sure, in the usual situation, it is anticipated that one will pray for the recovery of the patient. However, there are circumstances in which it is not only permissible but even commendable to pray for the death of the patient!

Rabbenu Nissim comments that a person is but human, and that while he is cognizant of the obligation placed upon him, he nevertheless may legitimately wish that the obligation had not been imposed. It is as if a person were to ask a friend to take care of some cherished possession, but the person assuming this responsibility finds the task too onerous, too burdensome, and hence asks of his friend, "Won't you please take your possession back? You watch over it; it is too hard for me to do so." But all the while the person making the request recognizes that, until it has been returned to the jurisdiction and domain of the rightful owner, his obligations as a bailee have not been extinguished.

If we recognize -- as we must -- that Judaism posits not only an obligation simply to rescue human life, but also an obligation to prolong human life and that this is part and parcel of the obligation assumed by means of acceptance of this Divine bailment, it becomes possible to understand more fully some of the exceptions that are built into that obligation. From the vantage point of Judaism, a physician certainly is charged with the alleviation of pain. Assuredly, he is charged with the obligation to restore patients to good health. But, as has already been stated, he is also charged with the obligation to prolong life. He is charged with that obligation because every moment of human life is infinitely valuable and infinitely sacred. He is charged with the maximization of human life quanta, if I may call it that. And, paradoxically enough, this leads to a very significant exemption from the general obligation to heal. Let me give you a case study, an actual example from responsa literature. Approximately a century age, someone approached a renowned Jewish authority and presented the following dilemma: There is a patient who is now on his death bed. If one does nothing, the patient will survive for a matter of weeks, not months, but weeks. In his black bag the physician has something that may be of help. There is a new drug available for use in a phase two experimental protocol. If the drug is administered and it works, the patient will be restored to good health; he will live to reach the proverbial three score and ten years of age and maybe even *biz hundert und tzvantzig* (till one hundred and twenty). But if the drug proves to be toxic, then it may well be the case that he will die within a matter of hours or, at the most, days. Is the risk warranted? Can the risk be justified as being consistent with Jewish law and morality?

What is the dilemma? We are confronted with a situation in which there are quanta of what I would call life-certain and these are measured against quanta of what I would call life-possible. The number of life-possible quanta that can be gained if the procedure is successful is greater than the number of life-certain quanta that are being risked should the procedure fail. The answer given by the authority to whom the question was put was that one should first consult with all physicians proficient in that disease who are to be found in the city. One should seek not only a second opinion, but a third and a fourth opinion as well, and then one should present both the majority and minority opinions to the *hakham she-ba-ir*, to the rabbinic authority of the city, for final adjudication. What is the point of all this? The Rabbi has not gone to medical school; the Rabbi has no experience in treating this illness; the Rabbi hasn't the foggiest notion regarding either the therapeutic properties or the toxic dangers associated with the drug in question. What in the world is one supposed to ask the Rabbi and how is he supposed to answer the question? I submit that there is a crucial component in any such decision that is not medical in nature and it is *that* matter which is submitted to a rabbinic authority for adjudication, viz., the question of the prudence of the procedure.

When one is dealing with a procedure that is inherently hazardous in nature, one is dealing with a situation that requires a prudent assessment of the risk-benefit ratio. In such matters Judaism and Jewish law recognize an area of discretion. Whenever the threshold level of danger has been met, the procedure is not mandatory. It is never mandatory because, unlike the cat who has the proverbial nine lives, man does not have an infinite number of lives to risk. Man has only one life and there are circumstances when one cannot risk its loss, even though the potential exists for a great return on the investment. There are certainly situations in which the possibility of profit is so limited that the risk must be regarded as imprudent, to say the least. In such situations the proposed course of action is not mandatory but is a permissible one. Just as it is permissible to take the risk, it is equally permissible to decline the risk because of the recognition that, while maximization of life-quanta is a definite value, it is precisely because every life-quantum is of infinite value that even one precious quantum of life need not necessarily be risked in anticipation of some greater return. Hence, it turns out that, while the physician is charged with prolongation of life and the maximization of these quanta of life, a hazardous procedure need not necessarily be undertaken. It may even be the case that a procedure that, from the perspective of medical science, may not appear to be terribly hazardous or risky may yet be regarded as hazardous in nature from the vantage point of Jewish law.

Part II: Patients' Issues

The notion of an experimental therapy and its non-obligatory nature is found in the writings of latter-day Jewish authorities. However, if one goes back to earlier sources, the notion of an experimental therapy is encountered, but in a somewhat different guise. The concept occurs in a context that, I think, is rather interesting. The Mishnah, *Yoma* 83a, refers to a person who has been bitten by a *kelev shoteh*, a "mad dog," which obviously must be understood as a dog that is afflicted with rabies. In antiquity, there was a remedy that was widely used and presumed to be effective with regard to rabies. The victim of a dog-bite was given a piece of what is described in the *Mishnah* as the *hatzer kaved*, apparently a lobe of the dog's liver, in order to ward off the disease. Since the dog is not a kosher animal the problem is obvious. Can an individual who has been bitten by a rabid dog and who is in danger of contracting that dread disease be treated in this manner? The first and most obvious reaction is: Of course, the victim may eat non-kosher food in order to avoid a fatal disease! It is a well-established principle of Jewish law that, with the exception of the three cardinal transgressions [murder, idolatry, and certain sexual offenses], all prohibitions are suspended in the face of danger. Rabies clearly presents a danger, a very serious danger, a clear and present danger, and hence all canons of Jewish legal logic would indicate that one should proceed to feed the victim a piece of dog liver if doing so will protect him against the disease. At least one of the Sages of the Mishnah, a certain R. Mattia ben Heresh, ruled that this was an entirely permissible procedure. But his colleagues disagreed. The majority opinion is that the victim may not be permitted to eat dog meat even if that is the only available remedy for rabies.

How is this position to be understood? Rashi (R. Shlomoh Yitzchaki) explains that the remedy was not a *"refu'ah gemurah,"* which I understand as meaning that the therapeutic power of this remedy had not been sufficiently established. Rambam (Maimonides), in his *Commentary on the Mishnah*, formulates a principle which casts further light upon the proper elucidation of this ruling. Permit me to quote Rambam's statement at some length because I find the language that he employs to be very instructive.

The Sages declare that one may not transgress the commandments other than in conjunction with a therapy, i.e., with regard to things which cure in accordance with nature. That is, a true matter derived by reason or experience that approaches truth. But to treat by means of things that cure by virtue of their *segulah* is forbidden because their power is weak, not [known] by virtue of reason and its [demonstrated efficacy on the basis of] experience is far-fetched; its advocacy by one who is in error is weak.

Rambam understood very well that not everything in medicine is known with absolute certainty, but he also understood that medical science can achieve at least an approximation of truth and that any putative cure not grounded in reason or experience cannot be regarded as scientific.

It is quite clear that use of an accepted scientific form of treatment is required even if there is no certainty that the remedy will either achieve a cure or eliminate the danger. No therapy is accompanied by a guarantee of efficacy. To the contrary, every therapy carries with it its own risk and dangers. In the words of Ramban (Nachmanides) in his *Torat ha-Adam*, "With regard to cures, there is naught but danger; what heals one kills another." Moreover, *Halakhah* (Jewish law) unequivocally specifies that its strictures are suspended even in situations in which success in preserving human life is only doubtful. The mere possibility of eliminating a threat to life suffices to set aside restriction of religious law.

Nevertheless, even "doubt" must be defined. Arguably, there must be a threshold level of anticipation of success below which the contemplated therapy cannot be deemed to be of even "doubtful" potential. A fervent hope that a cure may be obtained serendipitously cannot seriously be regarded as encompassed within the zone of doubt of which *Halakhah* takes cognizance. It is precisely the notion of cognizable doubt that *Halakhah* strives to elucidate in establishing the dichotomous categories that have come to be known as *refu'ah bedukah* and *refu'ah she-einah bedukah*. Whatever medicine has to offer on the basis of reason, experience, or experimentation that "approaches" or approximates truth is to be accepted. A remedy whose properties are not fathomed by reason or whose powers have not been confirmed by experience is described as a "*segulah*," a term that does not have a precise equivalent in the English language. Suffice it to say that a remedy whose scientific properties are not understood or which has not been tried and tested must be regarded as pseudoscientific. The chances that such a remedy will be effective are extremely remote and, accordingly, there is no reason to suspend the prohibition associated with eating the flesh of an unclean animal in feeding dog's liver to the bite victim in an attempt to treat a person who may be afflicted by rabies. This, I think, is the basis of the distinction between what in later rabbinic terminology is called a *refu'ah bedukah* and a *refu'ah she-einah bedukah*, between a therapy which is of known efficacy and a therapy which is of unknown efficacy.

The dichotomous categories of *refu'ah bedukah* and *refu'ah she-einah bedukah* must, however, be carefully delineated. The notion of known efficacy does not mean that the medication is accompanied by a gilt-edged guarantee that the medication will be effective in a specific instance and save the life of a particular patient. A *refu'ah bedukah* is to be understood as connoting a drug or other form of therapy that is known to be effective in at least some circumstances. Use of such a therapy, when medically appropriate, is deemed to be obligatory.

I believe that this provision of Jewish law is simply another one of the manifestations of the basic principle that man's obligations and responsibilities with regard to himself, his life and his body are the obligations of a bailee, an individual who has been entrusted with a valuable object for purposes of safekeeping and preservation. In terms of common law jurisprudence, a bailee is obligated to be diligent in preserving any object that has been entrusted to him for safekeeping. However, he is not obligated to employ any and every measure that might conceivably be of benefit in preserving the property that has been entrusted to him. To recast the same concept in Jewish law terminology, the obligation of a bailee is to preserve and to safeguard *"ke-de-natrei inshi"* -- "as people are wont to safeguard." With regard to bailments, the law establishes a prudent person standard. A bailee must act in a way that a prudent person would act in a similar situation. That is, he must act in the manner in which a person who indeed desires to preserve the object in question would act. However, the bailee is not obligated to pursue safety measures that go beyond the limits of prudence; nor is he obligated to take measures which are unknown, untried and untested in the hope that they may serve to protect and to preserve the object that has been entrusted to him. This, as I understand the matter, is the general rule to be applied in the treatment of all patients. Clearly, the most important application of this principle is in the treatment of the terminally ill. Modes of therapy that are mandatory must, of course, be provided on behalf of the terminally ill, but there may well be a desire to withhold nonmandatory treatment. On the other hand, it is entirely likely that all possible remedies will be used on behalf of a non-terminally ill patient -- including experimental procedures.

Let me hasten to stress that Judaism does not have one set of principles for treatment of non-terminally ill and another set of principles for the treatment of the terminally ill. Perhaps that is because Judaism recognizes that we are all afflicted with a terminal condition called "life." Nor does Judaism place any great emphasis upon a distinction between prolonging life and prolonging the process of death. That distinction is essentially a matter of semantics in which nomenclature is chosen to reflect a particular emotional predisposition. Since we want the diabetic to live, we speak of insulin as prolonging life; since we want the pain-ridden patient suffering from incurable cancer to die, we speak of placing such a patient on a ventilator as prolonging the process of dying.

From the vantage point of Jewish law, it is extremely important to recognize that a distinction between prolongation of life or prolongation of the process of dying is not very helpful in resolving the problems that confront us. One must, however, recognize that life is one long continuum which begins with the formation of genoplasm in the gonads and continues until there has been total decomposition of the body in the grave. Quite understandably, our obligations and responsibilities to the human organism are not uniform at all stages along this continuum. Rather, there exist differing obligations and responsibilities which vary in a manner appropriate to changes in the human condition along the various stages of the continuum. I have purposely referred to this entity as a "human organism" rather than as a "human being" because I am not at all concerned with when this organism becomes a human being and when the organism ceases to be a human being. Clearly, in Judaism, and I submit in any system of law or ethics, certain modes of behavior are regarded as appropriate with regard to this organism at any particular stage along this continuum and various other modes of behavior are regarded as inappropriate. The only questions which can be asked are, "Where are the lines of demarcation to be drawn along this continuum and what are the corresponding duties and responsibilities?"

Parenthetically, recognition of this principle serves to illuminate the matter of determination of death in Jewish law. The concept of death is not a scientific or a medical notion. The concept of death is, to be sure, a legal notion. It may be a metaphysical notion, and it certainly is a moral notion. The law must establish criteria for pronouncing death if it seeks to punish a person who causes the death of another or if it finds it necessary to provide for issuance of death certificates. Issuance of a death certificate merely certifies that the organism has reached a certain stage along this continuum at which a death certificate is appropriate. What ought to be the physiological criteria for issuing a death certificate? That is not a medical decision; that is an entirely different type of decision. The medical issue is limited to a determination of what can be done on behalf of the patient who manifests a certain clinical profile and to a determination that at a certain stage in his illness nothing further can possibly be done on behalf of the patient. The physician is uniquely qualified to provide details concerning the prognosis of a disease. The physician, and only the physician, can determine that a particular physiological state is irreversible. What type of treatment is appropriate under such circumstances is a question of an entirely different nature. Thus, for example, the issue of whether or not we should provide artificial nutrition or hydration for a person in a state of irreversible coma is a moral decision which must be made by a moral agent; the physician has no particular expertise or responsibility for making that type of determination. I do not wish to enter into a discussion of the question of the determination of time of death other than to say that it is the overwhelming consensus of rabbinic authorities that the classical common law definition of death accurately reflects Jewish tradition and is the only definition that can be accepted for purposes of Jewish law. Those criteria include total and irreversible cessation of all respiratory and cardiac activity and of all vital functions consequent thereupon.

Judaism certainly recognizes the notion of a *gosses*, defined roughly as a moribund patient, but then proceeds to define the physiological state in question in terms of very specific criteria. As a result, contemporary medical knowledge and technology may well nigh define the category out of existence. I do not want to enter into a detailed definition of the clinical state corresponding to *gessisah*; suffice it to say that we are clearly talking about a person in whom death is imminent. Moreover, it seems to me that the definition presented in the *Shulhan Arukh* contains two crucial elements: 1) The patient has lost control of bodily functions, including the ability to bring up phlegm or other secretions; and 2) the patient's condition is such that, *no matter what medical science can possibly do*, death will occur within 72 hours. Only when the functions of the human organism have deteriorated to the point that the patient is in such a state can the question of withholding treatment be entertained. Even so, it must be emphasized that if the downward physiological progression can be reversed, or even arrested, there is certainly an obligation to do so. To put the matter in only slightly different terms: If it is possible to reverse the state of *gessisah*, it is incumbent that this be done. However, if that state cannot be reversed, then medical obligations vis-a-vis the patient are somewhat different from medical obligations vis-a-vis other patients.

If you will permit me to use metaphorical and picturesque language, I will describe the underlying principle as follows: When the angel of death has entered the room, if you are fairly certain that you can take the angel by the scruff of his neck and throw him out, by all means do so. But, if you believe that you will be unsuccessful in expelling this angelic messenger from the room, then in interfering you will have succeeded only in hindering the angel in his ministrations. That is an exercise in futility. The principle seems to be: If you can't vanquish the angel of death, leave him alone. Please do not take these comments too literally. I am purposefully using picturesque language because I want to avoid language that distinguishes between prolongation of life and prolongation of the process of dying.

Moreover, these comments are an oversimplification of the obligations owed a moribund patient. Treatment of the *gosses* is one of the relatively few areas of bioethics in which there is significant disagreement between contemporary rabbinic authorities. That disagreement merely reflects a controversy that has existed for 150 years or so. Some authorities read the classic sources as indicating that there is only one difference with regard to the treatment of a moribund patient and the treatment of any other patient, i.e., that treatment in the nature of what Rambam categorized as a *segulah* may be suspended in the case of a *gosses*. The term *segulah* must be understood as referring to folk remedies, pseudoscientific treatment or attempts to harness spiritual or metaphysical powers in contradistinction to those modes of therapy which are of known and demonstrable efficacy.

The example which is given as a paradigm is that of a patient who is on his death bed and someone outside is noisily chopping wood. Rema (R. Moses Isserles), *Yoreh De'ah* 339:1, quotes *Sefer Hasidim* as declaring that the sound of wood-chopping prevents the soul from leaving the body.

This distresses the patient because the patient wishes to die. If the wood-chopping is stopped, the soul will be able to leave the body. Rema rules that, in the case of the moribund patient, it is perfectly permissible to interrupt the chopping of wood. This is virtually the only authoritative statement in rabbinic literature dealing with the treatment of moribund patients. A definition of the state of *gessisah*, for these authorities, yields but one result, viz., a means of determining that it is not necessary to continue to chop wood in order to keep the patient alive. Naturally enough, we chuckle at that result because we do not know of any causal relationship between chopping wood and keeping body and soul intact as a unitary entity. That is so because the chopping of wood and its interruption is no more than a *segulah*, a pseudoscientific measure.

It must also be remembered that, as explained earlier, the obligation to heal does not include an obligation to employ *segulot*, pseudoscientific or metaphysical measures. It seems to me that the majority of rabbinic authorities are of the opinion that only measures that may legitimately be withheld in the treatment of a moribund patient are those measures that need not be instituted in the first place, e.g., chopping wood or administering laetrile. For purposes of this discussion, I would label laetrile a kind of modern-day *segulah*. Laetrile yields no demonstrable scientific benefit. Laetrile is perhaps even a bit deleterious to the well-being of the patient, but I will ignore that for the moment. Assuming laetrile produces no detrimental side-effects, it certainly is not in the category of a *refu'ah bedukah*, i.e., a medicament of known and demonstrated efficacy. Administration of a *refu'ah bedukah* capable of prolonging the life of a patient is obligatory and, according to these authorities, cannot be removed even from a moribund patient.

Other rabbinic authorities maintain that interruption of wood-chopping is to be understood as a more general paradigm and hence withdrawal of any and all treatment from a moribund patient is to be sanctioned, provided that such withdrawal does not cause any additional pain to the patient. It must be emphasized that even those authorities agree that withholding of treatment is permitted only in the case of a moribund patient who manifests the physiological criteria of a *gosses*. My own impression is that this controversy is more theoretical than real because there are remarkably few patients who present a clinical profile corresponding to the *halakhic* criteria of *gessisah*, i.e., moribund patients who have lost control of bodily functions and of whom one can say with a reasonable degree of certainty that a majority of all patients in a comparable physiological state will die within a period of 72 hours, no matter what is done on their behalf. If the state of *gessisah* is defined in that matter, it becomes apparent that modern medical science has made such tremendous strides that patients satisfying those criteria turn out to be proportionally few in number. Moreover, patients who do satisfy those criteria are not the patients from whom physicians and family really want to withhold further treatment.

It should be added that there is an even smaller minority of rabbinic scholars who maintain that it is forbidden to initiate any medical treatment on behalf of a *gosses* if the patient is experiencing pain. However, since virtually all such patients are comatose that, too, is not a significant concern. The isolated statements of some rabbinic decisors to the effect that comatose patients also suffer pain must, I believe, be dismissed as based upon erroneous medical information.

One other matter with regard to which there is some controversy among contemporary rabbinic authorities is the withholding of treatment from a patient suffering excruciating pain. Unfortunately, this is an issue which has not received the detailed discussion it deserves. The few items that have been written with regard to this question are long on conclusions and rather short on sources, reasoning, and *halakhic* dialectic.

Let me try to present the issue as I understand it. There is an obligation not to stand idly by the blood of one's fellow (Leviticus 19:16), i.e., an obligation to save the life of a person who is in danger. However, an answer that is supplied by an early talmudic commentator is very significant for our discussion. The answer given by this authority is that the commandment, "And you shall love the Lord your God with all your heart, with all your life (*nafshekha*)" (Deuteronomy 6:5) is indeed understood by the Sages of the Talmud as meaning "even if He takes your life." This, however, serves to establish, not only the obligation of martyrdom, but also to establish the upper limits of martyrdom. One is obligated to sacrifice one's life, but one is not obligated to offer more than one's life. Withstanding torture, declares this authority, is a price greater than sacrificing one's life. Accordingly, he concludes, one is obligated to offer one's life rather than commit an act of idolatry, but one is not obligated to endure torture. It then follows that one is not obligated to suffer unspeakable, intractable pain -- the physiological equivalent of torture -- if that is the price that must be paid to preserve life.

In the real world, there is very little, if any, reason for a patient to suffer this degree of pain. It must be remembered that, to the best of all scientific knowledge, a patient in a comatose state does not suffer any pain whatsoever. For the noncomatose patient, pain medication may indeed compromise alertness and level of consciousness. Judaism, however, has no objection to rendering a patient unconscious if that is necessary to prevent pain. Morphine in doses sufficient to control severe pain may indeed suppress respiration, but Judaism has no objection to placing a patient on a ventilator if that is necessary in order to relieve pain. There is enough in the physician's little black bag to treat most forms of pain. Let me also state very briefly that heroin may also have a beneficial role to play in the management of pain. Some physicians maintain that heroin is not really needed at all; others claim that use of heroin is entirely appropriate and, in at least some situations, is the drug of choice in the management of pain. I honestly don't know which opinion is right and which is wrong, but I have a hunch. The Talmud tells us that the good Lord did not create anything in the universe without a purpose. If there is any purpose for heroin, it seems to me that it must be for the alleviation of pain. Therefore, I presume that there are some circumstances in which its use is totally appropriate. The problem is to convince the lawmakers. In Great Britain heroin may be prescribed by a physician for medicinal purposes and its use in the control of pain is quite legal. I have not heard any report indicating that medical use of heroin in England has been abused or that legalization of the medical use of heroin has made their drug problem any worse than ours. I would, therefore, certainly advocate the legalization of controlled substances for use in the treatment of terminally ill patients.

There is one other issue with regard to the treatment of the terminally ill that must be mentioned, namely, the general problem of truth-telling. Despite the emphasis Judaism places upon honesty in both word and deed, in some circumstances, Judaism not only permits, but encourages, lying. Judaism encourages lying when lying is therapeutic. A therapeutic lie is a *mitzvah* (commanded act). The best example of a therapeutic lie is the situation in which misinformation is given to a terminally-ill patient in order to enable him to believe that he is not terminally ill. Judaism would encourage such a fib on the general principle that one should make another person feel happy even if it is necessary to tell a white lie in order to accomplish that end. To adapt the classic example found in the Talmud: A wife comes home from a sale sporting a hat she has bought. The hat is nonreturnable. Her husband thinks the hat is hideous; he cannot stand it. If she discovers that her husband does not like the hat, she will be very upset. She will be offended that her spouse is disappointed in her taste and distressed that she has spent so much money only to become aggravated. What should the husband say to her? Judaism teaches that the husband should tell her that he loves the hat. And he should not let his conscience trouble him about the fib. That lie is justified simply to make a person feel good about himself or herself. But even more significantly, Judaism recognizes that disclosure to the patient that he is suffering from a terminal illness may itself hasten death. Since Judaism forbids any act that may hasten death, it teaches that one ought never tell people that they are terminally ill if such disclosure can possibly be avoided.

All this of course has a very serious impact upon the Jewish attitude toward hospices. The idea of a hospice is a beautiful concept. To quote the words of Rabbi Judah Ha-Levi in a different context: "The intent is acceptable, but the actions are unacceptable." The hospice is a wonderful idea; it is just the execution that is so terrible. I did not intend that as a pun, but it is a literal truth. The very use of the phrase "hospice" in addressing a patient is a form of execution. It announces to a patient who has any degree of sophistication that all who enter those portals shall not leave. That, in and of itself, is contrary to Jewish teaching. Moreover, if it is the accepted policy that a hospice will provide only palliative treatment and will not provide therapy even when, from a Jewish law perspective, therapy is indicated, the establishment of such a facility constitutes a violation of the ethical norms prescribed by Judaism. The notion that a medical facility ought to provide tender loving care in the finest sense of the term for a patient who is terminal is entirely laudable. That idea deserves to be applauded. It is the execution of the idea which leaves a lot to be desired.

Before AIDS came upon the medical scene, we were confronted with the prospect of having a significant surplus of hospital beds. Health-care administrators were concerned with the problem of what in the world they were going to do with all those beds. My bright idea at the time was that we ought to establish hospices within existing medical centers but not call them hospices. In such an institutional framework there would be no need to call them hospices. Hospice-like units could be set up to provide the best possible atmosphere and to provide everything that can possibly be provided for the terminally ill -- including appropriate therapy and certainly any and all appropriate forms of palliative treatment. But there is no reason to impart to such patients the message that there is no hope. The message to the patient should always be one of reassurance and hope.

I am well aware of the fact that Jews are not in a position to impose our views upon others even if we would wish to do so. But, by the same token, we should not shortchange ourselves. Unfortunately, we very often sell ourselves short because we do not recognize our proper role in God's plan for the universe. Rabbi Judah Ha-Levi aptly used a medical simile in depicting the role of the Jewish people in remarking, "As is the heart among the organs of the body, so is Israel among the nations of the world." The heart, in terms of its size, is a tiny, almost insignificant part of the total human organism, yet its physiological influence is profound, to say the least. As is the heart among the organs of the body, so is Israel among the nations of the world. In terms of our numbers, we are very small, a minuscule people. Yet, insofar as our potential ethical and moral influence is concerned, our influence is far beyond what we recognize it to be. We do have the potential for being a very, very potent and positive moral force. If only we would recognize our moral obligations and be sensitive to the fact that, by our own conduct and example, we can exert influence far, far beyond our numbers.

References

Bible. Masoretic text.

Babylonian Talmud. Vilna edition.

R. Judah he-Hasid. *Sefer Hasidim*. *Mekitzei Nirdamim* edition. Berlin, 5651-53.

Maimonides. *Commentary on the Mishnah*. Vilna edition.

Mecklenberg, R. Jacob. *Ha-Ketav ve-ha-Kabbalah*. New York, 1946.

Midrash Rabbah. Vilna edition.

Nachmanides. *Torat ha-Adam* in *Kol Kitvei Ramban*, ed. Charles B. Chavel, Vol. II. Jerusalem, 5723.

Shulhan Arukh. Vilna edition.

CHAPTER 12

THE CASE OF BABY M

Rabbi David M. Feldman, D.H.L.

I come to you from Teaneck, which is in the backyard, so to speak, of Hackensack, New Jersey. It is there that Judge Harvey Sorkow delivered his verdict in the famous case of surrogate motherhood and its implications for custody and paternity.

I have gone on record as deploring the outcome of the trial. Not necessarily the verdict in terms of custody, but the judge's summation, his *obiter dicta*, his charge to Mary Beth Whitehead. I feel he gave us a classic illustration of adding insult to injury: he injured her by "terminating" her parental rights and then insulted her with remarks about her character. I believe he ought at least to have added a word of commendation to her, on two counts. He should have thanked her for reminding us of the special bond of attachment that a mother forms with her child; and he should have gratefully acknowledged her message that surrogacy as an option ought to be discouraged.

To begin with, it must be said that the *Halakhic* problems are the least of it, the easiest to resolve. Some of the *posekim*, the decisors of Jewish law, had declared artificial insemination by donor -- the process basic to surrogacy -- to be adulterous; the progeny would then by definition be illegitimate. While Rabbi Yehudah Leib Zirelson, Rabbi Ovadiah Hadayah and others have so written, the majority of *posekim*, such as Rabbis Moshe Feinstein, Benzion Uzziel, Schwadron, Baumol and Walkin, ruled that adultery only occurs when there is a violation of marital intimacy, that it cannot be applied to a clinical procedure such as artificial insemination. If adultery is not involved, the child is legitimate; furthermore, the birth of such a child helps the donor father fulfill his *mitzvah* (commandment) of "be fruitful and multiply" (Genesis 1:28). Whereas a parent who adopts and raises a child does a great *chesed*, an ongoing kindness, by giving a child a home, only the parent who increases the number of children in the world by biological fathering, technically fulfills the Biblical commandment of *p'ru ur'vu* ("be fruitful and multiply"). This means that William Stern is fully the father of Baby M, and that Baby M owes him full *kibbud av* (paternal honor) under the commandment to honor one's father and mother (Exodus 20:12; Deuteronomy 5:16).

Baby M also owes full *kibbud em*, maternal honor, under the same commandment, to Mary Beth Whitehead. More important, she remains forever the daughter of Mary Beth in the genetic sense, which means that marrying any other of Mary Beth's children would constitute incest. In the related question of *in vivo* fertilization or host mother/embryo transplant, where there is a genetic mother and a birth mother, the debate involved even the U.S. Congress as to whether maternity is attributed to the mother who supplied the fertilized ovum or to the mother who lent her womb. Reasons for choosing the latter included the consideration that society "sees" the womb-mother giving birth; social order dictates attribution of maternity to her. On the other hand, the genetic mother gives the DNA, the repository of traits of genius or disease. No legal fiat or judge's decree can change that biological fact.

When the host mother, as in the case of Baby M, provides both the genetic and the gestational input, her maternity is doubly, triply strong. In the Talmudic imagery (*Kiddushin* 30b), "there are three partners in the creation of a child -- the father, the mother and God." Actually, the mother's contribution is more than the father's, if they are indeed quantifiable. Both parents offer genetic endowments, but the mother adds the nurture of the womb. Mary Beth Whitehead did not "carry" the child as one would carry, say, a package. She carried the child in the sense of symbiotic supply of nutrients and lifeblood. She endured morning sickness and the conscious and unconscious tending to the embryo's needs. And thus she bonded with the child profoundly. When a mother says to a recalcitrant or unappreciative child -- "Is that how you treat me after all I've done for you?" -- she probably has poignant reference to those nine months of "carrying."

Her right, therefore, to change her mind ought not to have been dismissed. The Talmud makes reference in another context to the difference in a woman's feelings for her child before or during the birth, and afterwards. A Talmudic passage (*Niddah* 31b) seeks and finds another reason for the Biblical provision that a woman after childbirth brings a sin-offering to the Sanctuary. The prosaic reason is obvious: a man or a woman must bring an offering to mark the completion of the purification period after physical discharges. But the Talmud offers a deeper reason: childbirth pain is severe; in pain she must have taken a vow never again to enter into pregnancy; the child is born, and in her joy she forgets both the pain and the vow; she forgets to have her vow formally nullified; hence the sin-offering! In cases of ordinary adoption, the birth mother has the recognized right to change her mind, for a period of time varying in various states. Here the contract of the natural father indeed makes a difference, and contracts are upheld on the basis of expectation. But there is no long-time history of surrogacy contracts for the husband to have developed that confidence, to protect him, that is, against her voiding the contract by returning the financial consideration. I regret that here the judge gave more weight to his expectation than to her maternal reality.

This is not to say that the judge was incorrect in the custody aspect of his decision. It may well be in the "best interests of the child" to be placed with the Sterns. It is noteworthy that Jewish law says very little about custody, leaving that primarily to the *shikkul ha-da'at*, the *ad hoc* prudential determination, of the judge. But even the fact that judgment was necessary, and took the family through so many months of public anguish, shows how the "best interests of the child" are invariably undermined by such an arrangement, and hence that surrogacy should not have been, by implication, encouraged in his verdict.

To leave the court decision and consider the basic issues, it must be said that Judaism is, in the modern phrasing, "pronatalist." That means that making possible a pregnancy and conception is a good thing, a *mitzvah*. To enable the couple to accomplish this end is to advance their religious and personal desideratum.   Hence, the Medical Ethics Committee of the Federation of Jewish Philanthropies of New York has made explicit what is implicit in Jewish law, namely that barrenness or infertility is an "illness," the absence of health. Contrary to the position of Blue Cross, according to which no reimbursement can be expected for fertility treatment, we regard infertility as no less a pathological condition than any other disorder. And the same mandate to heal, which bids us set aside conflicting ritual prohibitions and harness our energies to cure sickness, bids us do the same to overcome childlessness.

This mandate means that new technologies that assist in this objective are to be welcomed. Of course, Jewish law would never sanction recourse to such methods merely to spare one the inconvenience of pregnancy and childbearing, and certainly not in order to insure some package of genetic characteristics, such as blue eyes or tall stature.   But where the natural alternative is not available, medically-assisted ones become quite acceptable -- providing the *Halakhic* issues raised along the way can be resolved.

Artificial insemination is not to be excluded as a last resort. One of the first to officially sanction it, again in the absence of alternatives, was Rabbi Moshe Feinstein.   The procedure, he concluded, does not entail adultery and illegitimacy, but other problems do obtain. The uncertainty or concealment of paternity is the greatest of these, because unintentional incest could result.   The child born from such a procedure could unknowingly marry a sibling, a half-brother or half-sister conceived from the same donated sperm. Therefore, Rabbi Feinstein (*Igrot Moshe: Even HaEzer* 10) suggested in that original ruling (1961) that records of paternity should be kept and made available and, to render less likely the eventuality of incest, the donor should preferably be a non-Jew.   This latter provision was protested by other Rabbinic writers, so the former was emphasized (*Igrot Moshe: Even HaEzer* 2:11). Biological parentage should be on record and accessible to the principals in a possible marriage.

His cautionary wisdom has been vindicated on another score, that of donor insemination outside the sphere of surrogacy. In a study of the sources of sperm donation, it has been determined that a certain Midwestern facility attributed no fewer than 500 pregnancies from artificial insemination to one particular intern. A similar study found that 73 births resulted from the activity of one person in a Beersheba hospital. Aside from what this does to the health of the gene pool, the incestuous consequences of close in-marriage would be eugenically contraindicated.

Returning to surrogacy itself, other considerations give us pause. The Biblical precedent of Jacob and Bilhah and Zilpah is frequently cited, where these "bondwomen" were asked to conceive and bear alongside of Rachel and Leah (Genesis 30:3-5; 9-10). But there was neither artificial insemination nor the exchange of money in those Genesis narratives. More important, there was no custody question: Jacob, Leah and Rachel, Bilhah and Zilpah and all their children lived together in one household. No King Solomon was needed to have them sliced up or given away.

The exchange of money in this context troubles many of us. To stipulate a fee, beyond basic medical or legal expenses, is to engage in the buying and selling of infants, to do commerce with human subjects. Moreover, fees open the door to exploitation of the poor by the rich, to lure needy women to "rent a womb" for pay to the financially able sponsors. But my concern is not only with the monetary aspect; the practice bears similar dangers even when no money is involved. It can lead to a situation where psychological pressure may be felt by a fertile woman to bear a child for a sister or a friend, and worse, where an ongoing feeling of guilt is suffered by the woman who refrains from so doing. We are beginning to hear from surrogate mothers, in fact, who feel remorse for having relinquished a child because of or in spite of the fee, and from siblings who express their newly discovered vulnerability: if my brother or sister is negotiable, perhaps I am, too. There are all sorts of human factors beyond the legal and contractual that the Hackensack court has blithely overlooked.

Mary Beth Whitehead, by appearing to change her mind and return the monetary payment, has reminded us of the strong bond a mother feels for her natural progeny. But the duration of the trial, and her own plea that the practice not be encouraged, are an even more significant message to us. That surrogacy contracts not be honored is also the conclusion of the Warnock Commission in London two years ago. Other advances in reproductive technology are acceptable, it declared, but surrogacy leads to too many social and human complications. Australia has ruled out private as well as public agreements of this kind, and Israel seems to have done likewise. England's Chief Rabbi Immanuel Jakobovits (1984) readily agreed with that country's Warnock Commission, reiterating his moral condemnation of hiring a woman's body for this purpose. These and other dimensions of psychological and social detriment are coming to the surface in many places. This is what Rabbinic authorities meant when they said: even if technical adultery and illegitimacy are not involved, the family bond is shattered.

The family bond involves *yichus* in the best sense of that word. It means knowing one's parents and feeling the spiritual dimension of lineage, of advancing their values and aspirations, of giving and taking pride in family nurture and association. A child deserves an unfettered and undiminished sense of both parentage and lineage.

NOTE: Subsequent to this presentation, on February 1, 1988, the Superior Court of New Jersey overturned the ruling of the Hackensack Court. Without disturbing the custody decision, it restored Whitehead's maternal rights. Also, New York State, along with many others, prepared legislation voiding surrogacy contracts and negating legal and social advocacy of the practice.

References

Feinstein, M. (1961). Responsa *Igrot Moshe, Even HaEzer.*

Feldman, D.M. (1985). *Health and medicine in the Jewish tradition.* New York: Crossroad.

The Holy Scriptures. (1985). Philadelphia: Jewish Publication Society.

Jakobovits, I. (1984). *Human fertilization and embryology -- a Jewish view.* London: Office of the Chief Rabbi.

The Talmud. (18 vols.) (1961). I. Epstein (Ed.). London: Soncino Press.

CHAPTER 13

THE ACQUIRED IMMUNODEFICIENCY SYNDROME

(AIDS): JEWISH PERSPECTIVES

Fred Rosner, M.D.

Introduction

The response of society to the acquired immunodeficiency syndrome (AIDS) epidemic since the first cases were reported in 1981 has been interesting to observe. The medical community has been inundated with a veritable flood of books, journal articles and other publications on the medical, epidemiologic, viral, and immunologic aspects of the disease. The causative virus has been identified and characterized, and intensive efforts are under way to develop a vaccine.

The lay press is full of discussions of the social, political, economic and public policy issues relating to AIDS. Public hysteria has been fueled in part by the mass media and the nation's newspapers and magazines with sensational headlines such as "AIDS: A Time Bomb" and "AIDS - Can the Nation Cope?," and "AIDS Panic Disrupts American Blood Banks." As a result, some morticians refuse to touch bodies of AIDS patients, some children with AIDS are forcibly kept out of school, and some health care workers are avoiding contact with AIDS patients.   This fear of AIDS is totally unwarranted and often misinformed[1].

There are heated discussions about mandatory testing for antibody to the AIDS virus, now known as the human immunodeficiency virus (HIV). President Ronald Reagan in his first major speech on AIDS on May 31, 1987, ordered AIDS antibody testing of immigrants and federal prisoners and called for states to offer "routine" testing to marriage license applicants, people seeking treatment at sexually-transmitted disease clinics, and state and local prisoners. The Surgeon General of the United States, C. Everett Koop, M.D., called for AIDS virus antibody testing for all patients scheduled for major surgery.   According to a survey of state medical societies reported in the June 26, 1987 issue of the *American Medical News*, the majority of state legislatures had before them bills on mandatory testing and disclosure of test results. By early June 1987, more than 425 pieces of legislation on the subject of AIDS had been introduced in 47 state legislatures, though only about 20 had passed in 16 states. California, with 66 bills, was the state with the most legislation introduced. A California prosecutor proposed testing sexual-assault suspects for antibodies to HIV and filing charges - possibly even murder - against those who test positive. The initial impact of AIDS on public health law in the United States was summarized by Matthews and Neslund[2].

The defense department of the United States is testing the over two million members of the armed forces, and military officials will help health officials around the world to identify civilians exposed to AIDS by American military personnel.

An American Medical Association (AMA) sponsored conference was held in Chicago on April 21-22, 1987. At that meeting, Gary R. Noble, M.D., said that within five years there may be 50 million to 100 million people worldwide infected with the HIV virus, according to estimates of the World Health Organization (WHO). John Renner, M.D., asserted that there is an entire industry of disinformation, spreading panic and fear about the threat of AIDS. James H. Sammons, M.D., Executive Vice-President of the AMA, suggested that care for people with AIDS could be financed by placing a surcharge on the income of those infected with the AIDS virus. Also at that conference, Lloyd J. Kolbe, Ph.D., described a new federal plan for AIDS education that will help schools provide students with information to protect themselves from becoming infected with the HIV.

At the Third International Conference on AIDS held in Washington, D.C. on June 1-4, 1987, Jonathan Mann, M.D., director of the WHO's program on AIDS, stated that the AIDS epidemic has unveiled thinly-disguised prejudice about race, religion, social class and nationality. There is a rising wave of stigmatization directed against homosexuals, intravenous drug abusers, prostitutes, hemophiliacs, Africans in Europe and others, continued Dr. Mann. At that same conference, Anthony Fauci, M.D., director of the National Institutes of Allergy and Infectious Diseases, announced the beginning of clinical trials with an experimental antiviral drug, zidovudine (formerly known as azidothymidine, or AZT), in an attempt to prevent clinical AIDS from developing in asymptomatic seropositive people. On March 20, 1987, the Food and Drug Administration (FDA) granted approval for the new drug which had previously been shown to prolong survival time in AIDS patients with a history of *Pneumocystis carinii* pneumonia.

The ethical dilemmas posed by AIDS were discussed at length on the last day of the 1987 annual meeting of the American College of Physicians held in New Orleans. Some of these include the refusal of treatment that might be life-saving, decision-making in the case of incompetent homosexuals (family or lover?), withholding or withdrawing of life support systems, the cost of AZT and the availability of treatment, the role of physicians and other health care professionals in treating AIDS patients, confidentiality, privacy and much more.

The insurance industry is caught in a dilemma. It knows that homosexuals and intravenous drug abusers have a higher probability than others of contracting AIDS and could thus refuse to insure them and risk being charged with discrimination. Do insurance companies have the right to force applicants for life or health insurance policies to submit to testing for HIV antibodies? What is the proper balance between the individual's right to privacy and the insurance industry's right to know about life-style factors that can materially affect a person's chances of developing a disease? To what extent can, or should, the insurance industry shoulder the huge costs associated with catastrophic illness? There are no easy answers.

There are active sex-education programs being offered nationally, including the recommendations of no sex or safe sex, the latter by the use of condoms. Cardinal Joseph Bernardin of Chicago, addressing a plenary session at the above-cited AMA-sponsored conference on AIDS, stated that the normative way for living out one's sexuality is in a monogamous, heterosexual relationship of lasting fidelity in marriage. The Cardinal said he could not support the promotion of safe sex in educational programs seeking to curb the spread of AIDS. Meanwhile, the FDA has strengthened its inspection of condom manufacturers and repackagers and broadened its sampling of domestic and imported condoms in commercial distribution. The 1987 graduating class of the Harvard School of Public Health tossed condoms inscribed with "Ad venerem securiorem" (safe sex) to their classmates in celebration of graduation and as endorsement of the use of prophylactics in the fight against AIDS.

The global offensive against AIDS has spurred research and raised hopes[3]. On a nearly daily basis, new developments are being reported on the epidemiology, virology, immunology, transmission, prevention, clinical management, social and psychological aspects, and public policy, economic and legal issues. To date, there have been no major breakthroughs, just incremental increases in knowledge. Changes in human behavior have already occurred as a result of AIDS education. In the words of the Surgeon General, C. Everett Koop, M.D., the human immunodeficiency virus in many ways "spitefully remains a mystery."

Response to AIDS by the Jewish Community

The existence of Jewish patients with AIDS is well recognized. According to Dr. Harold Jaffe of the Centers for Disease Control in Atlanta, no one knows the actual number of Jews who are suffering from AIDS since such statistics are not recorded. Estimates range from several hundred to a thousand. In New York alone, more than forty members and friends of Congregation Beth Simchat Torah, the gay synagogue in Manhattan, have died[4]. The Chairman of the Board of that synagogue said at a meeting early in 1986 that he did not know even one rabbi he could call to counsel AIDS patients who asked him for help because of the fear and shame which make rabbis afraid to minister to such patients[5]. The gay synagogue in San Francisco, Shaar Zahav, has had several members of its congregation die of AIDS and has others who are now sick, according to Rabbi Yoel Kahn.

The same is true of Washington's gay and lesbian synagogue, Bet Mishpachah.

Until recently, "the response of Jewish religious, communal, and organizational workers ran from paralyzing ambivalence to enlightened action[6]." Early in March 1986, three of Judaism's four religious branches joined with gay and lesbian Jewish groups and a variety of Jewish organizations including the Rabbinical Assembly (Conservative), the Union of American Hebrew Congregations (Reform) and the Association of Jewish Family and Children's agencies in a task force to deal with the impact of AIDS on Jews[7]. The National Jewish AIDS Project, initiated by Daniel Najjar, its newly-named executive director, and Rabbi David Teutsch, executive director of the Federation of Reconstructionist Congregations and Havurot, became headquartered in Washington, D.C.[8]. Absent from the leadership are representatives of the Orthodox Jewish community. The project

> will seek to provide pastoral care and counseling of patients and their families by rabbis and Jewish social workers; visitation of the sick by *bikur cholim* committees, delivery of kosher food to patients at home and in hospitals; and proper burial services from Jewish funeral homes. In addition, it will serve as an advocate of increased funding for hospice and home health care programs, and civil rights protection for persons with AIDS... Special emphasis will be placed on outreach to both victims and their families[9].

Temple Beth Torah in Dix Hills, New York, during the first week of March, 1986, sponsored a symposium on AIDS[10]. Rabbi Marc Gellman, spiritual leader of the synagogue and organizer of the symposium, said it was important for the synagogue to have hosted such a community discussion. "The synagogue should not be centered on religious activities as narrowly defined but as broadly defined," he said. "The priests in the Bible were involved in identifying infectious diseases. To think that we care only about holidays and prayer is wrong. This is a community issue and one the synagogue ought to address."

The Jewish Board of Family and Children's Services in Manhattan held an open conference on AIDS in December 1985 and began providing services to AIDS clients and their families, Jews and non-Jews[11]. New

York's Federation of Jewish Philanthropies held a conference on February 6, 1986 dealing with the medical facts about AIDS and the resources being used to deal with it.   On March 26, 1986, a conference was held at the Central Synagogue in Manhattan about AIDS and the special needs of the AIDS population.   The following day, Federation's medical ethics committee, headed by Rabbi Moshe D. Tendler, conducted a symposium on the role of the family and society, as well as the religious implications of caring for AIDS victims.   On May 7, 1986, yet another Federation-sponsored conference was held that dealt in part with the theological implications of the disease.

In Baltimore, Dr. Lucy Steinitz, the executive director of the Jewish Family Service, implemented policy and training for her caseworkers and volunteers to handle AIDS victims[12].   Peter Laqueur is a gay Jew who directed HERO, the Baltimore-based Health, Education, Resource Organization that acts as an AIDS clearing house, providing resources for medical, financial and counseling needs.   Rabbi Mark Loeb of Baltimore's Beth El said of his congregants with sons who are gay: "It's a *mitzvah* to respond. We Jews, of all people, should understand pain and suffering. We need to be there for these people. We have a mandate to be there[13]." Rabbi Herman Neuberger of Baltimore's New Israel College noted that "no Jew in pain should be turned away.   Being a homosexual is one thing, but having AIDS is after the fact and we as Jews need to administer care and counseling."

At its semi-annual meeting in White Plains, New York in December 1986, the Union of American Hebrew Congregations called on every arm of the Reform Jewish movement to educate its 1.25 million members about AIDS and urged its member congregations to help deal with the nation's escalating public health crisis.   Rabbi Alexander Schindler, the Union's president, said to the 125 trustees:

> The challenge of our Jewish tradition is clear. Where there is illness and suffering, we must seek to comfort; where there is fear and prejudice, we must seek to dispel it with knowledge and education; where there is optimism and a commitment to life, we must seek to preserve the human spirit with hope and compassion.[14]

Schindler also reported on ways in which the organization was addressing the AIDS crisis.

Every Reform congregation in the U.S. and Canada received a packet of informational material about AIDS - including guidelines for counseling families of victims, names of local, regional and national support groups, hot lines and a suggested sermon - by early 1987.

Schindler announced that more than half of the organization's 13 regional offices will include workshops on AIDS at their forthcoming biennial meetings and that a cadre of rabbis and lay persons in each region would be trained to furnish counseling support and leadership on the subject.

Educational programs on the disease will be developed for use in the movement's adult education courses and for its youth division through its religious schools, summer camps and publications for young people, Schindler said.

He also told the trustees that AIDS would occupy a major place on the agendas of the spring convention of the Central Conference of American Rabbis (the Reform rabbinical organization) and the Union's fall biennial in Chicago, and so it did.

In Israel, the Health Ministry set up blood testing centers around the country to test for HIV antibodies. Although AIDS is not common in Israel, the testing of all donated blood insures the lack of transmission of the disease to recipients of blood transfusions.

Homosexuality and Drug Abuse in Judaism

Ninety percent of all patients with AIDS are homosexuals or intravenous drug abusers. The Bible labels homosexual intercourse as an abomination (Leviticus 18:22) and ordains capital punishment for both transgressors (Leviticus 20:13). This biblical directive is codified by Maimonides[15].

The biblical, talmudic, and rabbinic views on homosexuality, lesbianism and bestiality are discussed in detail by Preuss[16], Lamm[17], and Freundel[18]. Lamm states that homosexuality, in at least some forms, should be recognized as a disease, and this recognition must determine our attitude toward the homosexual. Judaism allows for no compromise in its abhorrence of homosexuality, sodomy, lesbianism and bestiality, but encourages both compassion and efforts at rehabilitation. We must offer medical and psychological assistance, concludes Lamm, to those whose homosexuality is an expression of mental aberration, who recognize it as such, and are willing to seek help. We must be no less generous to the homosexual than to the drug addict, to whom society extends various forms of therapy upon request.

Freundel[18] posits that Jewish law views the homosexual or drug addict no differently than it does a Sabbath desecrator or an adulterer who has no greater or lesser rights or obligations. He deserves no special treatment or concessions nor any special vilification. The Jewish community should deal with the practitioner of homosexuality as a full-fledged Jew, albeit a sinner. He should be counselled and treated and be the concern of outreach and proper education. Freundel disagrees with Lamm who, while condemning the act, removes culpability from the homosexual and views him as an individual forced by heredity and/or environment into a biblically-forbidden activity. Freundel concludes that

> Judaism rejects the suggestions that homosexuality is either a form of mental illness or an "acceptable alternate life-style." Judaism's position would be a third and as yet unconsidered option. Homosexuality is an activity entered into volitionally by individuals, who may be psychologically healthy, which is maladaptive and inappropriate...our task is to treat and redirect this individual to more appropriate and fulfilling activity.

Judaism's view of consciousness-expanding drugs such as LSD has been discussed by Brayer[19] who evaluates the personality changes claimed by LSD from a psychological viewpoint, and the validity of religious claims from the *weltanschauung* of Jewish law and Jewish thought. The harmful effects of marijuana are one of the reasons to prohibit its use[20]. The same can be said about tobacco smoking[21]. Certainly the abuse of narcotics and other substances by intravenous and other routes is detrimental to one's health and, therefore, prohibited in Judaism. The Torah tells us not to intentionally place ourselves in danger when it states *take heed to thyself, and take care of thy life* (Deuteronomy 4:9) and *take good care of your lives*

(Deuteronomy 4:15). The avoidance of danger is exemplified in the Bible in the commandment to make a parapet for one's roof so that no one fall therefrom (Deuteronomy 22:8). Hence, the smoking of cigarettes and marijuana and the abuse of intravenous narcotics, acts which constitute a definite danger and hazard to life, are considered pernicious habits and should be prohibited. The subterfuge of "it is no concern of others if I endanger myself" is specifically disallowed by Maimonides[22] and Karo[23] in their legal codes.

Jewish Legal Questions Relating to AIDS

Two essays[24-25] discuss in detail a variety of *halachic* (Jewish legal) questions pertaining to AIDS. Since most patients with AIDS are homosexuals and/or drug addicts, they are considered sinners, thereby raising the following questions: Should a Jewish drug addict who develops AIDS as a result of sinful activity be treated any differently than any other patient? Should the Jewish homosexual who develops AIDS as a result of "abominable" behavior be treated? Does Judaism teach compassion for all who suffer illness irrespective of whether or not the illness is the result of practices which Judaism abhors and prohibits? Should every effort be made to heal these patients or at least alleviate their pain and suffering? Is a physician or nurse or other health worker obligated to treat a patient with AIDS or other contagious disease if there is a risk that they may contract the illness from the patient? Should the Jewish community expend resources for AIDS research and treatment since most such patients are sinners? Would not the resources better be allocated to the health of law-abiding citizens? Can patients with AIDS be counted in a quorum of ten men (*minyan*)? Can they serve as cantors or Torah readers? Should they be given honors in the synagogue? Can a *kohen* (priest) with AIDS offer the priestly blessing (*duchan*)? Can a patient with AIDS serve as a witness in a Jewish legal proceeding? Is a patient with AIDS to be given all the usual burial rites? Is mourning to be observed for such a patient?

For an in-depth *halachic* analysis of these and other questions relating to AIDS, the interested reader is referred to the two above-cited essays. Briefly, Jewish law treats AIDS as it would any other health issue. According to Freundel[26], the crucial concern is the severity and degree of danger. As contact with an AIDS patient may present some medically undefined level of danger, individuals have the right to be concerned for their own health. Other individuals may choose to ignore the risks and trust that God will protect them. Health professionals, concludes Freundel, are duty bound to have a modicum of faith in God and they must competently and professionally minister to AIDS patients.

I have previously pointed out[27] that while homosexuality is characterized in the Torah as an abomination, we are nevertheless duty bound to defend the basic rights to which homosexuals are entitled. The Torah teaches that even one who is tried, convicted and executed for a capital crime is still entitled to the respect due to any human being created in the image of God. Thus, his corpse may not go unburied overnight[28]. The plight of Jewish AIDS victims doomed to almost certain death should arouse our compassion.

In Judaism, the value of human life is infinite. Whether a person is a homosexual or not, we are obligated to give him proper care if he is sick, charity if he is needy, food if he is hungry, and a burial after death. If he breaks a law of the Torah, he will be punished according to the transgression. Even if AIDS is a punishment by God for the sin of homosexuality, Jewish tradition teaches us that such a divine affliction may serve as an atonement for that sin or the patient may repent while ill, making the AIDS victim even more deserving of our mercy and lovingkindness as a fellow Jew.

The compassion of Jewish law in requiring treatment for AIDS patients, however, should not be confused with acquiescence in the behavior of homosexuals who develop AIDS. Under no circumstances does Judaism condone homosexuality, which the Torah characterizes as an abomination. Nevertheless, the patient with AIDS should be treated and his life saved. To stand idly by and see the homosexual die without trying to help him is prohibited[29]. Evil should be banned but the evildoers should be helped to repent[30].

Conclusion

The acquired immunodeficiency syndrome (AIDS) has been described as this century's greatest health peril. Thousands have already died from the disease and there is no cure in sight. The medical, epidemiologic, viral and immunologic features have been well described and the causative virus identified. Attempts at prevention of the disease by developing a vaccine; screening of all blood, organ and semen donors; and educating high risk groups to change or avoid behavioral risks have been slow, in part because of under-funding and legal issues of constitutional rights. The emotional toll on patients with AIDS, their families and their caregivers needs to be actively and aggressively addressed. The public hysteria should be alleviated by a well planned, coordinated and implemented educational program involving not only health professionals, but the mass media which have in part fueled the public fear about AIDS. Prudent practices in the health care and private industry work places have been suggested and should be followed. Public policy decisions need to be made with compassion and understanding.

The Jewish community has responded to the AIDS problem. Clear Jewish legal statements have been made about the rights of AIDS patients to be treated, the obligation of health professionals to treat them and the need to overcome not only the medical aspects of AIDS, but to treat the psychosocial and religious deviations from normally-sanctioned Jewish behavior which may have led, in some instances, to the development of the disease. May the Divine Healer speedily cure all His people from the ravages of AIDS and all other diseases!

References

[1]Friedland, G.   Fear of AIDS.   *New York State J. Med.* 1987; 87: 260-261.

[2]Matthews, G.A. and Neslund, V.S.   The initial impact of AIDS on public health law in the United States - 1986.   *J.A.M.A.*   1987; 257: 344-352.

[3]Marwick, C.   Global offensive against AIDS spurs research and raises hopes. *J.A.M.A.* 1987; 258: 11-12.

[4]Elliott, R.   Jewish AIDS care program launched.   *The Jewish Week*, March 7, 1986, p. 5 and 46.

[5]Deutsch, J.S.   Jews with AIDS: Community faces a tragic new challenge.   *Long Island Jewish World*, March 7-13, 1986, p. 3 and 13-14.

[6]*Ibid.*

[7]Cohler, L.   New national group formed to help Jews hit by AIDS. *Long Island Jewish World*, March 7-13, 1986, p. 10.

[8]Elliott, *op. cit.*

[9]*Ibid.*

[10]Ain, S.   Health expert: AIDS spreading at slower rate.   *Long Island Jewish World*, March 7-13, 1986, p. 11.

[11]Ain, S.   N.Y. Jewish groups mobilizing to meet AIDS crisis.   *Long Island Jewish World*, March 7-13, 1986, p. 12.

[12]Jacobs, P.   AIDS, a Jewish problem, too.   *Baltimore Jewish Times*, July 11, 1986, pp. 60-63.

[13]*Ibid.*

[14]Anonymous. Reform body launches AIDS program. *The Jewish Week*, Dec. 12, 1986, p. 10.

[15]Maimonides, M. *Mishneh Torah, Hilchot Issurey Bi'yah* 1:41.

[16]Rosner, F. (transl). *Julius Preuss' Biblical and Talmudic Medicine.* New York, Hebrew Publ. Co., 1978, pp. 490-500.

[17]Lamm, N. Judaism and the modern attitude to homosexuality, in *Jewish Bioethics* (F. Rosner and J.D. Bleich, eds). New York, Hebrew Publ. Co., 1979, pp. 197-218.

[18]Freundel, B. Homosexuality and Judaism. *J. Halacha & Contemp. Society* #11 Spring 1986, pp. 70-87.

[19]Brayer, M.M. Drugs: A Jewish view, in *Jewish Bioethics* (F. Rosner and J.D. Bleich, eds). New York, Hebrew Publ. Co., 1979, pp. 242-250.

[20]Feinstein, M. Responsa *Iggrot Moshe, Yoreh Deah*, Section 3, #35.

[21]Rosner, F. *Modern Medicine and Jewish Ethics*, Hoboken, N.J., Ktav and Yeshiva Univ. Press, 1986, pp. 363-375.

[22]Maimonides, M. *Mishneh Torah, Hilchot Rotze'ach* 11:4 ff.

[23]Karo, J. *Shulchan Aruch, Choshen Mishpat* 427 and *Yoreh Deah* 116.

[24]Freundel, B. AIDS: A traditional response. *Jewish Action*, Vol. 47, #1, Winter 5747/1986-87, pp. 48-57.

[25]Rosner, F. AIDS: A Jewish view. *J. Halacha and Contemp. Society.* No. XIII, Spring 1987, pp. 21-41.

[26]Freundel, *op. cit.*

[27]Rosner, F. *J. Halacha and Contemp. Society. loc. cit.*

[28]Deuteronomy 21:23.

[29]Leviticus 19:16.

[30]Psalms 104:35.

CHAPTER 14

REFLECTIONS ON THE PATIENT'S QUESTIONS:

WHY ME?   WHY NOW?

Clarification of the Questions:
H.J.C. Swan, M.D.
Rabbi Levi Meier, Ph.D.

Reflections:
Lord Immanuel Jakobovits, Ph.D.

Dr. Swan:

"Why Me? Why Now?" There is always a "me," and there is always a "now," in terms of life and death, because that is the nature of man. Within these larger questions, however, there are questions that arise daily on the issues of "when" and "how."

Several case examples may serve to illustrate my point. The first case has to do with an elderly lady who had a history of hypertension and atrial fibrillation for approximately 40 years. She also had a tendency not to consume animal products of any sort, and as a result she developed a severe calcium loss and osteoporosis and was disabled in terms of her mobility. She developed a relatively moderate stroke and I saw her at that time. The prognosis for the stroke was excellent. However, in the course of her subsequent illness, it became obvious that because of her bone disease, she was unable to rehabilitate. I saw the patient again, a week or two later, and we agreed that further major intervention was not warranted. The patient lingered for a while and then died. As a physician, I had absolutely no worry about what was done and that it was the right thing to do for a lady of 93. As her son, it was quite different, because she was my mother.

There is an excellent and relevant commentary in Ecclesiastes 3: "To everything there is a season, a time for every purpose under heaven. A time to be born and a time to die"... "A time to weep"... "and a time to mourn." It was very easy for me, as a son, to think sad but wonderful thoughts about a very wonderful person who had an immense impact on my life. She was difficult from time to time, unforgiving from time to time and hypercritical most all of the time. Even when I was 60 years of age, she clearly regarded me as some rather unruly child. But that's okay too.

However, another case was, for me, much more difficult. It involved a relatively young man, 44, who moved from New York to Los Angeles to run a successful savings and loan institution. I met him through my church, the Hollywood Presbyterian Church. At the time that I got to know him, he had three children, and he was looking for a home. He was doing all of the things that people who have just moved do. We were meeting socially on a weekly basis, and at the second or third meeting, he said, "You know I have not been feeling well; I have to go to a doctor." I saw him the next week and he said, "I was seen by this doctor and he referred me to another doctor," and he named one of our most prominent oncologists. I saw him one week later, and already the weight loss had set in, and in two weeks he was dead. With fulminant cancer involving the liver, the lung, the stomach and the pancreas, his system was just overwhelmed. That case put me in mind of "Why Me? Why Now?" This relatively young man, in the prime of his career, was cut down, and I could not find anything in Ecclesiastes to explain it.

However, this case brought to mind an extraordinary incident about which I heard in 1981. At that time I was in Durban, South Africa, at the Wentworth Hospital, the teaching hospital of the Medical School.

Wentworth is a non-white medical school. Half of the medical school students are Indian and half are Black, mostly Zulus, because the Zulu tribes live in that part of Natal, South Africa. It was at Wentworth that I heard the following story.

One of the bright Zulu resident doctors had brought his father to the hospital for abdominal complaints. The diagnosis was liver cancer, and the father -- a Zulu chief -- subsequently died. The autopsy, which revealed the course of the disease, was seen by the son. The body was then shipped back to the tribal lands, and the son came to his supervisor and requested a week of absence which was immediately granted. The supervisor said, "What are you going to do, where are you going to go?" The young man -- a trained physician -- said, "We have to find out why he died." Tribal practices involve the use of a witch doctor, to ferret out *who* put the disease in the patient. This young man was going to go and participate in that practice, which usually results in the deaths of two or three others, usually the enemies of the ruling faction, who are then placed in the grave with the deceased. The supervisor replied, "Well you saw the autopsy, you understand what happened. Why are you doing what you are doing?" The young Zulu doctor turned around and said, "Can you tell me who put the cancer in my father? How did it get there?" I think that if I were to put that question to any other physicians, they would be pretty much stuck to come up with an answer.

In our concept of knowledge, we try to examine at least three issues: the natural sciences, which is the relationship of man to nature; law, the relationship of man to man; and theology, the relationship of man to God, God being to many a concept, perhaps, rather than a specific entity. God is something within and without oneself, something that is totally different from any of the other aspects of life. We have to turn from the natural sciences, within which medicines lies, and from the law, to theology. That area encompasses what we should want to know and what we want to guide us regarding how we should behave from the standpoint of ethics and morality in general.

I will remember forever a remark made by Victor Frankl some years ago. He said that "Many people deny a God, our God or the concept of God, but I have never met anybody who did *not want* there to be a God."

For moral and theological wisdom we turn to the Lord Jakobovits.

Rabbi Meier:

I am asked "Why Me? Why Now?" every day in almost every patient's room, though the form of the question may vary somewhat. Sometimes the patient will say to me, "Yesterday, I was in a concentration camp and today I had a mastectomy." Or, "Yesterday I lost a child," -- referring to 30 years ago -- "and today I am undergoing bypass surgery." In the patient's mind, the sequence of time is not 30 years or 25 years or 45 years. Patients see these events as sequential, and they ask the questions, "Why Me? Why Now?"

The Lord Jakobovits:

For me, the topic of "Why Me? Why Now?" is a great challenge. I must have given literally thousands of lectures on the impact of Jewish teachings on the practice of medicine, and above all the moral problems that arise with the spectacular advances of medicine in our times. However, this is the first time that I am faced with a rather new challenge, dealing with what is primarily not so much a moral or an ethical or religious issue, but rather what I might term a pastoral issue. The selection of this topic was made by Rabbi Meier. This choice reflects his sensitivity to the special needs of patients encountering catastrophic illness. Indeed, my esteemed colleague is rightfully regarded as the pioneer of Jewish pastoral medicine.

I was greatly intrigued by the words of Dr. Swan, such a distinguished practitioner of the medical arts. The cases that he presented encapsule the areas that I feel I might comment on, because they hold the key to my response. The first case concerned his mother. The truth is that no two individuals are alike. Every individual is different. You cannot give one answer that can satisfy a variety of individuals, because we all encounter this problem of "Why Me?" and "Why Now?" in a highly individual way. No one answer will satisfy numbers of people. In other words, the answer must be tailored to the person who asks it. Whether it is a mother or it is any other individual, we are all unique, and therefore, there cannot be a generalized answer.

The case of the Zulu doctor also illustrated to me a cardinal point. Dr. Swan pointed out that any physician would probably be stuck for an answer if asked who put the cancer into the Zulu tribesman. Physicians have no answer, and I would not be honest if I did not state that rabbis also have not got an answer. These questions have been asked over the ages, in the Book of Job and by numerous philosophers, thinkers and theologians, yet no one has come up with a definite answer. I want, first of all, to very honestly share the limitations of my own understanding, my own knowledge, and my own certainties in an area that is full of perplexities and full of unanswerable questions. I can share a few thoughts on the subject, although they are not necessarily answers.

First, one must make a fundamental distinction between these questions being asked before one gets ill, when the questions are hypothetical, and when the questions are asked after tragedy has struck. The answer that can be given theoretically to healthy people is one thing; the answer that can be given to those who actually experience suffering is something entirely different.

Furthermore, these questions can seemingly be multiplied a million times. Don't we ask, "Where was God at the Holocaust?" There were six million people, innocent men, women and children, struck down in the most fearful of all persecutions and mass murders in human history. So we could multiply the questions "Why Me?" and "Why Now?" a million times, and we would still not know the answer. The questions are no different, whether they regard one individual or a million. A new term, "Holocaust Theology," has been coined in an attempt to cope with the problem of "Where was God during the Holocaust?" The question of "Where was God during the Holocaust?" is no different from the question of "Where was God?" when there occurs a sudden infant death. A little innocent child, months old, is suddenly discovered by the mother to have expired; no prior symptom, no reason, no sin, no punishment, no theology behind it. One can ask exactly the same questions, "Where was God? Why Me? Why Now?" Just as there is no ultimate answer to the Holocaust, there is no ultimate answer regarding this stricken baby. What can one tell the parents? In other words, the questions raised by suffering are not multiplied by the number of people who undergo such suffering. You cannot multiply infinity. The grief is infinite, whether it is for one human being or six million human beings.

One of the best known words in the whole of our literature is the word *Echa*, meaning *why* or *how*. The Book of Lamentations is called *Echa* in Hebrew. The question of *Echa* was what we asked nationally; we challenged God and we did not receive an answer. When we lament, we cry out to God and we say "*Echa*." We do not ignore the problem, and we do not, in a superficial way, suggest that we have all the answers.

I must also mention the need to see these questions in perspective. As rabbis, we occasionally notice that someone new has turned up at daily services, in a great state of agitation. This person might have someone in his family who has been stricken with serious illness, so in his despair the man comes to the synagogue and asks the rabbi to recite a prayer for a child, a wife, or a parent who is seriously ill.   Strangely it very rarely happens that people come to the synagogue on a sudden urge occasioned by joy, because they have been fortunate in business or things have gone exceptionally well for them. One ought to go and not only render thanks to God, but also ask God, "Why Me? Why Now?" Why did I deserve to have this good fortune? What have I done to be favored by providence? In other words, we are biased. When misfortune strikes, we challenge God. When fortune strikes, we do not ask such questions. Similarly, in the case of the six million, we ask, "Where was God?" What we do not ask with equal passion is why we were saved. After all, but for the almost sheer accident of our parents or grandparents escaping from Europe, we would not be here. Every one of us would be reduced to a speck of dust on the blood-soaked soil of Europe. Yet, by a stroke of extraordinarily good fortune, we are among the saved remnant, and we ought to ask, "Why Us?" and "Why Now?" Why are we here now when others, by the millions, have been done to death?   We cannot be selective and outspoken only when we have complaints, yet keep silent and be unresponsive when the situation is reversed, when "Why Me?" and "Why Now?" refers to good fortune and to blessings.

My late, revered father, of blessed memory, who was a very experienced rabbi, once told me that there are two things which we humans want more than anything else. Number one is, we want to live. Who wants to die? Number two, we want to know the future. However, my father added, if these two wishes were granted, it would be the greatest curse that we could experience. Because if we could live forever, we would never get anything done. We would not need to do something today or next year.

We would have hundreds of years to wait. We could never be productive or creative in life if we knew it was timeless. Moreover, if we suffered from any worry or anxiety, there would be no end to it. We would know that we could never be relieved of that suffering. So my father said, "You see how short-sighted we human beings are. We ask for life because we want to live forever; yet if God would grant this wish, it would be our biggest curse. The second thing that we ask for involves a similar dilemma. We want to know the future. Yet, if we had this knowledge, it would be a curse for us."

Imagine that the six million Jews who were done to death in the Holocaust had known twenty years earlier what lay in store for them. They could not have lived for those twenty years either. The fact that the veil is drawn over our vision of the future is the greatest blessing. Imagine if people with some dreadful cancer had known years earlier what lay in store for them. They could not have lived for those years either, if they had the definite knowledge of what their condition would be. Therefore, the greatest blessing that God gives us is that we do not know the future. We must realize that we do not know what to ask for, because what we ask for could be the greatest curse that God might give us. There is a certain subjectivity here, in which we misjudge and misgauge that which is in our ultimate interests.

There is also another aspect of suffering that must be addressed. We, as Jews, do not sanctify or idealize suffering. We do not believe that there is a virtue or a value in suffering. On the contrary, we believe it is a curse and we should do whatever we can to overcome and resist it. For instance, it would have been inconceivable in the Jewish tradition for us to object to the discovery of chloroform as an anesthetic in childbirth. In the last century in Europe, when chloroform was first presented to relieve the birth pains of the mother, it was resisted by some other faiths for theological reasons. Since God had said, "In pain shall you bear children" (Genesis 3:16), what right did one have to fly in the face of providence? It was not until Queen Victoria employed chloroform for the birth of her own royal children that it became accepted. To us Jews, there is no virtue whatever in going through the pain of giving birth if it can be avoided with the use of chloroform or today's far more effective means.

Maimonides similarly argued that we are entitled to resort to medicine and to mechanical contrivances to make life easier. He states that surely one can apply the plow to the field in order to sow seeds and bring forth produce, although this act flies in the face of providence. One might think that even this type of intervention should not be allowed, since "by the sweat of thy brow shalt thou eat bread" (Genesis 3:19). If we were to idolize suffering as a virtue, then we should not be allowed to make life easier by either using medicine to overcome illness or using technical contrivances to overcome the toil and hardship of winning bread out of the soil. We do not believe in this approach. We believe that, on the contrary, we should use our God-given human ingenuity in order to ease life and to overcome the pangs of suffering and the ordeal of winning our bread. We should avoid suffering by using any means that are available to us. The value lies not in suffering. The value, as we see it, lies in how we face suffering, how we respond to the challenge of suffering.

Some seven years ago I appeared on a BBC television program in Britain which dealt primarily with genetic counseling. When people are afflicted with a serious genetic disease, facing the problem of having a seriously ill child, how do you counsel and how do you respond? We were then dealing particularly with Tay-Sachs, which is a hideous disease, from which the child will invariably die within the first years of life. I said that we recognize and will not argue that this situation is an unmitigated disaster and tragedy. We must do our best to stretch out a healing hand and to provide a word of comfort, as well as communal facilities that will ease the lot of parents having to cope. But, I added, in many cases such suffering can ennoble. It can bring forth from the heart of the parent, or of the supporting staff, the nursing staff, or the social service staff certain virtues that would otherwise remain hidden. There can be people who become nobler people, finer people, more virtuous people because they have had such an experience. I have heard this response from parents themselves. Some parents have told me that grievous as the experience was, it made them more refined, it made them more sensitive to the suffering of others and more aware of the blessings that they have received from their other children who are perfectly normal.

After I made the comment that suffering sometimes helps to ennoble people, I took questions from the phone-in service of the BBC. Most of those who phoned in were people who had had to deal with their own stricken children. Some said that they could not find anything noble in suffering; they were devastated and there was no redeeming feature for them. But the majority who phoned in said yes, Rabbi, you said something that we always sensed somehow but could not quite articulate. Yes, we feel we are better human beings, more refined, more sensitive human beings than we were before this child was born. We feel that a dimension has been added to the refinement of our hearts, sensitivities that would otherwise have been blurred and we would not have experienced. That child of ours, who went through all of this and put us through all the ordeals and died so young, added a new dimension to our humanity.

This account is not meant to sanctify suffering but to acknowledge that the effects of suffering can be ennobling and can turn us into better human beings. Who can better testify to this truth than we, the collective Jewish people, who are the historic people of suffering? We believe that suffering has made us into a people that sometimes feels more, senses more, shares more and has greater empathy because we know what suffering is and can therefore appreciate the suffering of others. When we went out of Egypt after the ordeal of hundreds of years of slavery, after our babies were drowned in the Nile, we were told not to abhor the Egyptians. Although they inflicted all the suffering on us, we were told not to treat them in the way we were treated, because we were strangers in the land of Egypt and therefore know the lot of the stranger. Consequently, forever we must look after strangers in a proper manner that we as Jews ought to know best. These behaviors are based on the knowledge of what it means to be a stranger and what it means to be persecuted. Though there is no direct answer to "Why Me? Why Now?," perhaps we can find some positive by-products of suffering that can help make us into more worthy human beings, so that we can contribute more to society. Perhaps we can become a little more caring, identifying a little more with the suffering of others, thereby helping to make a better world.

We are essentially a people with uncrushable optimism. If we were not we would not be here. We have said, collectively and individually, in the words of the Psalmist, "Though God has tried us sorely and afflicted us, He has not left us to die" (Psalms 118:18). In other words, we preferred a life of suffering to a death with glory, where we had the choice. We could have had a death with glory at any time in our history. All that we needed was a certificate of baptism and we could have lived like everyone else, with all the freedoms and all the equality.   We preferred to have our convictions and to suffer for them.   If we did not enjoy the freedoms and blessings of life, our children might, or our grandchildren might at some future date.   And so we survived.   We are here to tell the story, and we now have a State of our own.   We enjoy a degree of affluence that is perhaps unparalleled in the whole of our history, and freedoms that we enjoy because we have persevered, we have held out.   We have never been prepared to accept the verdict that there will be a final solution.   There is nothing final about our lives; we carry on.

Let us apply that attitude to the individual as well.   There is a beautiful saying in the Talmud (*Berakhot* 10a) that even when a sharpened knife is placed at your throat about to cut you, do not despair, even at this stage.   God will help you, will save you, will rescue you; you will survive. Therefore, we have a life-affirming optimism, which we will not easily surrender.   We will not undermine the belief that we will make it.

It is *most* essential in any pastoral treatment to maintain the rays of hope, because part of the therapy is that hope.   A person with hope has greater resources of spirit and of body to resist the afflictions of suffering. Some call it psychosomatic medicine, though its name makes no difference. Hope itself is a therapy, and therefore, one ought to communicate as well as possible that degree of hope that does not easily surrender to despair.

Selected English Bibliography on
Jewish Medical Ethics

Abraham, S.A. (1980). *Medical halachah for everyone.* New York: Feldheim Publishers.

Bleich, J.D. (1977 and 1983). *Contemporary halakhic problems.* The Library of Jewish Law and Ethics, Volume IV and X, (N. Lamm, Ed.). New York: KTAV Publishing House, Inc., Yeshiva University Press.

Bleich, J.D. (1981). *Judaism and healing: Halakhic perspectives.* New York: KTAV Publishing House, Inc., Yeshiva University Press.

Feldman, D.M. (1974). *Marital relations, birth control and abortion in Jewish law.* New York: Schocken Books.

Feldman, D.M. (1986). *Health and medicine in the Jewish tradition.* New York: Crossroad.

Feldman, D.M. & Rosner, F. (Eds.). (1984). *Compendium on medical ethics.* (6th edition). Federation of Jewish Philanthropies of New York.

Goodman, R.M. (1979). *Genetic disorders among the Jewish people.* Baltimore: John Hopkins University Press.

Gribetz, D. & Tendler, M.D. (Eds.). (1984). Medical ethics: The Jewish point of view. *The Mount Sinai Journal of Medicine*, January-February 1984, *51*(1).

Jakobovits, I. (1975). *Jewish medical ethics: A comparative and historical study of the Jewish religion attitude to medicine and its practice.* New York: Bloch Publishing Company.

Meier, L. (Ed.). (1986). *Jewish values in bioethics.* Max Martin Salick Memorial Lectureships. New York: Human Sciences Press.

Preuss, J. (1978). *Biblical and Talmudic medicine.* (F. Rosner, trans.). New York: Sanhedrin Press, Hebrew Publishing Company.

196

Rosner, F. (1972). *Modern medicine and Jewish law.* New York: Yeshiva University Department of Special Publications.

Rosner, F. (1977). *Medicine in the Bible and the Talmud.* The Library of Jewish Law and Ethics, Volume V, (N. Lamm, Ed.). New York: KTAV Publishing House, Inc., Yeshiva University Press.

Rosner, F. (1984). *Medicine in Mishneh Torah of Maimonides.* New York: KTAV Publishing House, Inc., Yeshiva University Press.

Rosner, F. (1986). *Modern medicine and Jewish ethics.* New York: KTAV Publishing House, Inc., Yeshiva University Press.

Rosner, F. & Bleich, J.D. (Eds.). (1979). *Jewish bioethics.* New York: Sanhedrin Press, Hebrew Publishing Company.

Rosner, F. & Tendler, M.D. (1980). *Practical medical halacha.* New York: Rephael Society, Association of Orthodox Jewish Scientists, Feldheim Publishers.

Index

About the Editor

Levi Meier, Ph.D., is Chaplain at Cedars-Sinai Medical Center and a psychologist in private practice in Los Angeles, CA. He received his M.S. in gerontology and Ph.D. in psychology from the University of Southern California. Rabbi Meier was ordained at Yeshiva University, where he received an M.A. in Jewish Philosophy. Through his varied and extensive clinical and educational background, he serves interchangeably as rabbi, psychologist, gerontologist and thanatologist. This is the third book in his series on Jewish values. The first two are entitled *Jewish Values in Bioethics* and *Jewish Values in Psychotherapy*. He is also Special Issues Editor of the *Journal of Psychology and Judaism*.

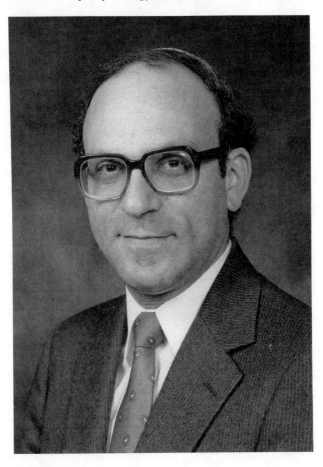